DARWIN'S WORMS

DARWIN'S WORMS

ADAM PHILLIPS

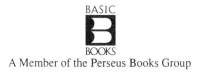

BASIC

BOOKS

A Member of the Perseus Books Group

First published in Great Britain in 1999
by Faber and Faber Limited

Copyright © 2000 by Adam Phillips

Published by Basic Books,
A Member of the Perseus Books Group

Photoset by Wilmaset Ltd., Wirral

Library of Congress Cataloging-in-Publication Data
Phillips, Adam.
  Darwin's worms / Adam Phillips.
    p. cm.
  Includes bibliographical references (p.) and index.
  ISBN 0-465-05676-8
  1. Darwin, Charles, 1809–1882—Contributions in
philosophical anthropology. 2. Freud, Sigmund, 1856–1939—
Contributions in philosophical anthropology. 3. Philosophical
anthropology—History—19th century. 4. Philosophical
anthropology—History—20th century. I. Title.

BD450 .P5112 2000
128—dc21
                                                    99-088832

01 02 03 04 / 10 9 8 7 6 5 4 3 2 1

to E.P.

This man loved earth, not heaven, enough to die.
Wallace Stevens, 'The Men That Are Falling'

Nature too will not remain supernatural.
Arthur Hugh Clough, diary entry, 15 July 1848

Science presupposes that what is produced by scientific work should be important *in the sense of being 'worth knowing'. And it is obvious that all our problems lie here, for this presupposition cannot be proved by scientific means.*
Max Weber, *Science as a Vocation*

Happiness is something entirely subjective.
Freud, *Civilization and Its Discontents*

Contents

Prologue

Nature is but a name for excess.
William James, *A Pluralistic Universe*

John Cage tells the story somewhere of going to a concert of music composed by a friend of his. The composer had also written the programme notes for the music in which he said, among other things, that he hoped his music might go some way to diminishing the suffering in the world. After the concert his friend asked him what he thought of the event and Cage answered, 'I loved the music but I hated the programme notes.' 'But don't you think there's too much suffering in the world?' the friend asked, obviously put out. 'No,' Cage replied, 'I think there's just the right amount.'

Everyone is shocked by how much suffering there is in the world, as if we really believe there could, or should, be much less. Indeed, talking about justice or scientific progress are both ways of talking about potentially avoidable suffering. We need to believe that someone can intervene in our suffering and make a noticeable difference. If this unavoidable fact of the excess of unhappiness in the world could once provoke a loss of religious faith – how could a God worth worshipping allow so much misery, indeed victimize his own son? – it now tends to create a more helpless kind of dismay. After all, in a secular

3

world who can we blame but ourselves, or nature? Religious despair has turned, that is to say, into political despair. God can no longer redeem us, and political process cannot sufficiently protect, or even represent, the people and things we most value; global capitalism can make democracy seem amateur, while the only potent religions are fundamentalist in intent.

From a political point of view – one that takes economics, and therefore exploitation, seriously – Cage's story is horrifying. It seems to expose the callousness, the heartlessness, of smart Zen: Cage as merely compulsively idiosyncratic, doing his shock therapy on his friends. And yet for some people who believe in something they often call nature, usually without a capital letter – people like Darwin and Freud and their followers – there is a sense in which there is just the right amount of suffering in the world, even though there is still too much. Both these writers are obsessed, in one way or another, by the kinds of suffering that, in their view, no living creature can escape. To be alive, they tell us, let alone conscious, is to be subject to certain unavoidable pressures, is to be ineluctably involved in conflict. And they both seem to want us to believe that while political systems may modify our suffering, they can never significantly diminish it. To be in nature – and now there is nowhere else to be – demands, they imply, a more realistic acknowledgement of the limits of politics, of what we can do to improve our condition. Ostensibly sceptical about political action, they seem to encourage a politics organized around, essentially mindful of,

4

what in their view politics cannot change. Even though for their critics – and often for themselves as critics of their own work, as secret sharers of their own words – their writings are, whatever else they are, politics by other means. When they warn us of the dangers of our own utopian (or redemptive) longings, they also offer us their own preferred worlds. In their descriptions of human nature, they want to give us a sense of realistic possibility.

'Nature,' Raymond Williams wrote, 'is perhaps the most complex word in the language.' It is used to justify both politics of diverse persuasions and the apolitical. It becomes the repository at once for everything deemed to be essential about ourselves and for everything considered to be most troubling; our foundation that is also our antagonist. In this conceptual muddle – that is the legacy of a theological world view – nature can seem to be at once the problem and the solution. If in the old world the drama was between God and nature, with 'Man' (as we were then called) as the middle-man, completing or failing to complete the triangle, then we can see Darwin and Freud as among the people involved in taking God out of the picture, leaving us with nothing between us and nature. If there is nothing outside nature, it becomes nonsensical to talk of nature, and especially human nature, as being divided against itself. Nature is, as it were, always on its own side. So when people are destructive, or self-destructive, they are not acting against their own nature, they are just being natural in ways we don't like. Instead of talking about the natural and the unnatural – or even nature and culture – we can talk about the parts of nature we prefer and why we prefer them.

But with the advent of secular science, to say something was natural became a rhetorical (though not always less truthful) way of saying that something was inescapably important, and that we had no choice in the matter: that nature effectively set some kind of limit to what we might think of as politics (our attempts to change the world by acknowledging, and conciliating where possible, rival claims). If it is 'natural' for people to be competitive and avoid pain and death; if it is 'natural' for children to be brought up by two parents of the opposite sex; if it is 'natural' for us to understand ourselves and others – then this is where certain kinds of discussion stop, and we must bear our fate. Nature replaces consensus or law or duty as our guide. Nature dictates what is worth talking about. It seems most persuasive, in other words, to appear to be speaking on nature's behalf. As though at the end of the day nature tells us what to do.

Darwin and Freud as naturalists – as great natural history writers – radically changed our sense of what was worth talking about, and therefore our ways of talking. After reading their work people couldn't help but be suspicious about what they themselves believed, and how they had come to their beliefs. Darwin and Freud made it very difficult for us not to use a certain kind of vocabulary when we refer to ourselves; words like sexuality, competition, childhood, the past, became compulsory in our self-descriptions. And they made us wonder, by the same token, what people who are writing about nature and human nature are actually writing about; whether, that is to say, we can tell the descriptions from the prescriptions.

Their work was scandalous because it disfigured people's cherished ideals, and so compelled people to revise their hopes for themselves. Havoc was played with people's priorities, but always with the implicit assumption that such redescriptions could change people for the better; that if we ditched redemption, say, or dreams of perfect happiness or complete knowledge, or took our histories more to heart, we might be more happily in this world rather than any other one. But this involved, on the one hand, simply taking for granted that certain kinds of suffering were just part of life, built in to what it is to be a human being; and, on the other hand, wondering in new ways why transience had always been so daunting. Their stories about suffering, that is to say, were stories about our relationship to change. They wanted to convert us to the beauty of ephemera.

Because of the Oedipus complex, Freud's mythic account of human origins and development, desire is what ensures our survival, while at the same time being fundamentally forbidden (we depend on our parents, but they are experienced as 'belonging' to each other, and therefore as also taboo). So from a psychoanalytic point of view it is the neurotic's project – 'neurotic' being Freud's scientific jargon for an ordinary person – to ensure that he has the right amount of suffering, because he is unconsciously guilty about his natural, i.e. unavoidable, desires, and therefore requires punishment (crime without punishment means the world falling apart). And the individual suffers more simply just because she desires, and desire entails conflict and frustration. In Darwin's view, to be in nature – not, that is to say, divinely endowed: not believing there is anywhere else to be – is to be in a war dominated by scarcity of resources and potential extinction. Conflict, and therefore anguish and unease, are integral to their sense of what life is like.

Both writers describe our bodily lives – and for both a life is synonymous with a body – as astonishingly adaptive and resilient, but also excessively vulnerable, prone to many deaths, and shadowed by the reality of death. Notably obsessed by what Frank Kermode called 'a sense of an ending', they are preoccupied by remains, by evidence of and from the past. Masters of retrospect, they distrust prophecy; they insist that the present never catches up with the past, and that the past tells us nothing reliable about the future.

For Darwin the primal struggle to survive and reproduce obviously entails avoiding that terminal disappearance called extinction (extinction being the death of the species and so the death of deaths). Darwin is haunted by irredeemable loss. 'Domestic varieties (of animals),' he writes, in a sentence that would have been resonant for Freud, 'when turned wild, *must* return to something near the type of the original wild stock, *or become altogether extinct.*' The curious emphasis here of his italics makes it sound like an order, just as the phrase 'altogether extinct' (like being a bit pregnant) has the nonsense of fear in it. It is starkly either/or: adapt or die; and the adaptation itself, even if successful, involves suffering the loss of previously successful adaptations.

'The individual,' Freud wrote in one of his last notes, just months before his death, 'perishes from his internal conflicts, the species perishes in its struggle with the external world to which it is no longer adapted.' If his reflections on the species are patently Darwinian – and perhaps the 'species' is also the Jews whose fate so much preoccupied him towards the end of his life – his sense of the individual's end is distinctively his own. Freud's wish – understandable if only in terms of his fleeing from the Nazis to 'die in freedom' in London – is that the individual die from within: that his death should not be inflicted from outside, that the internal world should hold sway over the external world. For Darwin the struggle was to survive in order to reproduce and thereby sustain the continuity of the species. For Freud the struggle, as we shall see, was to satisfy oneself, and essential to this satisfaction was to die in one's own way: from inside, as it were. There was the unavoidable suffering of conflict; but there was the pleasure of 'dying in one's own fashion', something, Freud asserts, that we might even suffer in order to be able to do.

Freud at his most fantastically speculative proposed, late in his work, that there was a death *instinct*. The death instinct – that, Freud writes, 'represents the greatest obstacle to civilization' – is, like Freud himself, not overly impressed by civilization. Because our lives are driven by the wish for satisfaction, they are a chronicle of losses; but they are also driven, Freud maintains, by a peculiarly destructive part of ourselves, by the wish to die. And yet this fictional death instinct – something of an artist itself – seems to want a particular, personalized death for us. For Freud, as for Darwin, there is not just the right amount of suffering in any conventionally moral sense of right: for who could ever condone suffering? But there is a necessary amount. Our instincts, at once the source of our suffering and of our satisfaction, ensure the survival of the species and the death of the individual.

The amount of suffering in the world is not something added on; it is integral to the world, of a piece with our life in nature. This is one of the things that Freud and Darwin take for granted. But it is one thing not to believe in redemption – in saving graces, or supernatural solutions – and quite another not to believe in justice. So the question that haunts their writing is: how does one take justice seriously if one takes nature seriously? Neither Darwin nor Freud is politically polemical in his writing, and they are both, as I have said, sceptical about political solutions to the problems they saw in life (and neither man took kindly to his ideas being taken out of what he decided was their appropriate context). They were, in their own terms, scientists not social reformers; and science could seem like a legitimate refuge from politics and the other more apparently sordid forms of investment that made up the world they worked in. If science is for us one of the forms political life can take – by definition, a vested interest – we have to try to remember that Darwin and Freud thought of themselves as trying to tell the truth about nature, and nature was what the truth was about. One could only understand human life by understanding its place in nature. And the three truths they took for granted about 'Man' were: that Man is an animal, that he must adapt sufficiently to his environment or he will die, and that he dies conclusively. They both declared, in different ways, the death of immortality. After the death of God it is transience that takes up our time. Nature is careless with 'her' creations. She is endlessly fertile, but to no discernible end. One couldn't, that is to say, believe in Nature in the way that one could believe in God. To talk about justice now would be to talk, one way or another, about adaptation; about the ways in which we want to get on with all the natural phenomena that make up our environment (the history of psychoanalysis comes down to a debate about the nature of adaptation). Whatever it is now that sustains life – and it is stories about what keeps life going (in both senses) that Darwin and Freud keep telling us – does not seem to care about its quality. Suffering is only a problem for us.

And yet to think of Darwin or Freud as pessimists is

too crudely reassuring. They are only pessimists compared to certain previous forms of optimism (the belief
in redemption, or progress, or the perfectibility of
Man). We are not merely trapped in what they call
nature: we are also released into it. The despair, the
horror and the disillusionments they suffer in their
discoveries and their inventions make them seek their
own new-fashioned consolations and satisfactions. We
read them, that is to say, for their redescriptions of
happiness; for what they find to celebrate. In Darwin's
lifelong interest in earthworms, and in Freud's lifelong
antipathy to biography, we can find what they found
to praise. And it was bound up, as we shall see, with
the place they gave to death, and therefore to transience, in our lives. In their notes from underground
they are not seeking stays against time. They are
unseduced by monuments.

'The brilliance of the earth is the brilliance of every
paradise,' Wallace Stevens wrote; and one can only
write the poems of the earth, as Darwin and Freud did,
if one is happily convinced that there is nowhere else to
go. When transience is not merely an occasion for
mourning, we will have inherited the earth. And it
was at inheriting the earth – making sense of our lives
as bound by mortality not seduced by transcendence,
by after-lives – that they both worked so prodigiously.
They want to teach us to let time pass. But inheriting
the secular earth required a sense of history, not merely
leaps and bounds of faith. It required forms of knowledge and methods of enquiry that didn't need to exalt
themselves, as though they were alternative religions.

12

Clearly the new languages of Darwin and Freud have been immensely influential. Their versions of nature – that is to say, their versions of what we are really like – have had a pervasive influence. A lot of people now think of childhood and sexuality as the sources of their suffering, just as many people tend to think of themselves as virtual animals struggling competitively for survival. What we inherit from the past is now a cultural obsession; and the nature of inheritance itself informs our most compelling fictions. Whether or not we read Darwin and Freud, they read us; we speak a version of their languages. We can't easily forget what they wanted to persuade us was true. Their stories are still difficult to get round. And they were both preoccupied, throughout their writing lives, by the ends of life, in both senses: its purpose, and the place of death, and even of extinction, in the ways we live – by death as the exemplary fact, the fact that lures us into fictions.

For Darwin the story to tell was how species can drift towards extinction; for Freud, as we shall see, the story was of how the individual tended to, and tended towards, his own happiness and his own death. In each case it is a death story that uniquely illuminates the life story; indeed, that makes it intelligible. What makes creatures die is deemed to be a key to how they live (as if you can only start telling the story when you know what is driving it to its conclusion). Whether any given species was aiming to avoid extinction in order to reproduce, or whether any individual was driven to die in her own way as some kind of consummate satisfaction, the pragmatic implication was clear. If death was at once final and unavoidable, it was also a kind of positive or negative ideal; it was either what we most desired, or what, for the time being, had to be avoided at all costs. For both Darwin and Freud, in other words, death was an organizing principle; as though people were the animals that were haunted by their own and other people's absences (birthdays remind us that we were once inconceivable). Modern lives, unconsoled by religious belief, could be consumed by the experience of loss.

So what else could a life be now but a grief-stricken project, a desperate attempt to make grief itself somehow redemptive, a source of secular wisdom? Now that all modern therapies are forms of bereavement counselling, it is important that we don't lose our sense of the larger history of our grief. It was not life after death that Darwin and Freud speculated about, but life with death: its personal and trans-generational history. 'We demand,' Ruth Anna Putnam writes, 'that our image of the world be hospitable to our most urgent interests.' It is the consequence, if not always the intention, of both Darwin's and Freud's writing to make our lives hospitable to the passing of time and the inevitability of death, and yet to sustain an image of the world as a place of interest, a place to love.

Redemption – being saved from something or other – has been such an addictive idea because there must always be a question, somewhere in our minds, about what we might gain from descriptions and experiences of loss. And the fact of our own death, of course, is always going to be a paradoxical kind of loss (at once ours and not ours). But the enigma of loss – looked at from the individual's and, as it were, from nature's point of view – was what haunted Darwin and Freud. As though we can't stop speaking the language of regret; as though our lives are trailed by disappointment and grief, and this in itself is a mystery. After all, nothing else in nature seems quite so grief-stricken, or impressed by its own dismay. And it was, unsurprisingly, in our experiences of loss that we might feel most abandoned in a world without God; radically inconsolable in such a starkly natural world, the bearers of a gloom apparently unshared by any other creatures. How could it be possible that we were only natural creatures, but that nature was felt to be insufficient for our needs? Either nature must be in some (old-fashioned) sense evil, or we have misconstrued our needs.

Darwin and Freud showed us the ways in which it was misleading to think of nature as being on our side. Not because nature was base or sinful, but because nature didn't take sides, only we did. Nature, in this new version, was neither for us nor against us, because nature (unlike God, or the gods) was not that kind of thing. Some of us may flourish, but there was nothing now that could promise, or underwrite, or predict, a successful life. Indeed, what it was that made a life good, what it was about our lives that we should value, had become bewildering. The traditional aims of survival and happiness, redescribed by Darwin and

Freud, were now to be pursued in a natural setting.
And nature seemed to have laws but not intentions, or
a sense of responsibility; it seemed to go its own
unruly, sometimes discernibly law-bound, way
despite us (if nature was gendered as a mother, she
was difficult to entrust ourselves to; and if we could
love a mother like this, what kind of creatures were
we?). And though we were evidently simply parts of
nature – nature through and through – what nature
seemed to be like could be quite at odds with what or
who we thought we were like.

Nature, apparently organized but not designed, did
not have what we could call a mind of its own,
something akin to human intelligence. Nor does
nature have a project for us; it cannot tell us what to
do, only we can. It doesn't bear us in mind because it
doesn't have a mind ('One is inclined to say that the
intention that man should be happy has no part in the
plan of creation,' Freud writes, knowing that there is
no plan and no creation). And what we called our
minds were natural products, of a piece with our
bodies. So we couldn't try to be more or less natural
– closer to nature, or keeping our distance from it –
because we were of nature. It was not like a place we
could leave, but only, perhaps, a place we could find
out more about. As though we might be more at home
in nature once we realized what kind of home it was
(or, indeed, whether home was the right word for
these particular living conditions). This, at least, is
the implicit hope in what Darwin and Freud have to
tell us: that what we are living in – what we cannot

help but live with – can be made more than bearable by their descriptions of it. Whether we are 'survival machines' (in Richard Dawkins' phrase), or 'desiring machines' (in Deleuze and Guattari's phrase), or not like machines at all, it's worth construing what we are like; it's worth going on with the analogies. If, once, we could think of ourselves as (sinful) animals aspiring to be more God-like, now we can wonder what, as animals without sin (though more than capable of doing harm), we might aspire to.

Darwin and Freud, as we shall see, are notably sceptical about what was once called the 'perfectibility' of Man. Indeed, for both of them we are the animals who seem to suffer, above all, from our ideals. Indeed, it is part of the moral gist of their work not merely that we use our ideals to deny, to over-protect ourselves from, reality; but that these ideals – of redemption, of cure, of progress, of absolute knowledge, of pure goodness – are refuges that stop us living in the world as it is and finding out what it is like, and therefore what we could be like in it. Darwin and Freud, that is to say, give us their versions of reality – that they call nature, and by implication human nature – in order to persuade us to reconsider our hopes for ourselves.

We have been looking, they suggest, in the wrong place, for the wrong things; spellbound by ideas of progress and self-knowledge only to discover not that, as we already knew, such things were difficult and demanding, but that they quite literally did not exist, and didn't give us the kinds of lives we wanted. That we have been hunting for unicorns when our energies might have been better spent. That the one pleasure we have denied ourselves is the pleasure of reality (what Freud called the 'reality principle' wasn't merely – or solely – the enemy of pleasure, but its guarantor). And if we are to take Darwin and Freud seriously as writers, we have to acknowledge the ways in which reality was a viable term for them: that they used the word to do something. Because, as a concept, it was a synonym for nature, it was rarely ironized by them. Reality referred to what we were diminished by refusing to acknowledge.

Pursuing his 'enquiry concerning happiness' in *Civilization and its Discontents*, Freud writes of

the three sources from which our suffering comes: the superior power of nature, the feebleness of our own bodies and the inadequacies of the regulations which adjust the mutual relationships of human beings in the family, the state and society. In regard to the first two sources, our judgement cannot hesitate long. It forces us to acknowledge those sources of suffering and to submit to the inevitable. We shall never completely master nature, and our bodily organism, itself a part of that nature, will always remain a transient structure with a limited capacity for adaptation and achievement. This recognition does not have a paralysing effect. On the contrary, it points the direction for our activity. If we cannot remove all suffering, we can remove some, and we can mitigate some: the experience of many thousands of years has convinced us of that.

It is such acknowledgements, not their disavowal, that point us in the right direction; it is the realities of nature that are our best source of inspiration. Nature becomes another word for what is actually possible. And psychoanalysis for Freud was to help us distinguish – as does politics – the inevitable from the chosen. To recognize how adept we can be at stunting our energies.

By the end of the nineteenth century finding out what people were like entailed finding out through scientific methods – in all their surprisingly various forms – what nature was like. For increasing numbers of people 'Man's' relationship with God and with justice was subsumed by this project. Darwin and Freud thought of themselves as discovering the facts about nature and human nature. They were not, in their view, providing scientific foundations for their political convictions, but what would be, by definition, the foundations of any political system. For Darwin the nature his science had revealed was a 'war' that he described as a process of natural selection. Freud's nature was a war between his mythical life instinct and death instinct. Freud's common word for the fundamental nature of human nature was 'instinct' (or the drives, or the 'id'). And he writes about the workings of instinct in human beings, as opposed to other animals, as especially obscure. When he writes about nature explicitly, he stresses that 'she' will never be completely mastered by 'Man'; and he tends to describe her as awesome and vengeful ('With these forces nature rises up against us, magnificent, cruel, implacable.'). Since we ourselves are natural – made of nature's forces – Freud, like Darwin, can't seem to get away from an absurd image of 'Man' as the animal who is always trying to master what he has always already been mastered by.

It was inevitable that these new versions of nature would complicate traditional moralities. Conflict, chance, survival, reproduction, the family, sexual satisfaction and death were newly minted words in these stories, quickly shedding some of their more familiar associations. Darwin and Freud had produced scientific and quasi-scientific redescriptions of nature as continual flux. There was no longer such a thing as a relatively fixed and consistent person – a person with a recognizable identity – confronting a potentially predictable world, but rather two turbulences enmeshed with each other. If through increasingly sophisticated scientific experiments a new nature was emerging, this new nature was revealing that lives themselves were more like experiments than anything else. Though Darwinism and psychoanalysis did not come out of the blue – indeed, it was integral to both theories that nothing came out of the blue, that everything has a history if not a cause – they were still shocking, judging by the virulence of the response they provoked, and continue to provoke. History, natural history, had become the most transgressive of disciplines.

But if we take Freud's fiction of unconscious desire (his idiosyncratic version of instinctual life), and Darwin's fact of natural selection, what are we actually left with, what have they left us to be going on with? Clearly not any kind of licence for amoral competition or sexual permissiveness. Nor indeed any straightforward endorsement of, or prescription for, specific ways to live. As how-to books their works are especially (and revealingly) unpromising. And this is for a very simple reason: nature, as they describe it, is law-bound, but human nature is radically unpredictable, puzzling to itself. If there are laws of human nature, some of them at least are of a peculiarly recondite logic. And just knowing about evolution – or believing in unconscious desire – doesn't tell us what to do (next). The sense we can make of ourselves is as nothing, they imply, compared to the powers that have made us what we are.

In Darwin's terms, our descriptions of ourselves are always survival-driven and circumstantial; and circumstances are always changing. From Freud's point of view unconscious desire, by definition, renders us only minimally intelligible to ourselves (and often, only sensible in retrospect, when it may be too late). The fact that we want to survive and reproduce, and the fiction that we desire in the way Freud describes, tells us remarkably little about how we should live. Indeed, it tends to ironize prescription (when it doesn't render it cynical). And yet, of course, Darwin and Freud furtively prescribe in their writing through what they praise. Their morality resides in their celebrations, as much as in their dismay: where they find beauty is where they find happiness; their prejudices are cover stories for their ideals. When Darwin writes about God, or when Freud fulminates against biographers – those traditional, and notorious, authors and plotters of other people's lives – they are telling us, in their own ways, about the kind of world they can genuinely believe in, the kinds of life stories that make sense to them.

'That there is much suffering in the world no one disputes,' Darwin wrote in his *Autobiography*. 'Some have explained this in reference to Man; by imagining that it serves for his moral improvement. But the number of men in the world is as nothing compared with that of all other sentient beings, and these often suffer greatly without any moral improvement.' We suffer, Darwin implies – as Freud will, but for different reasons – also from moralizing our suffering. And it is by comparing ourselves with other 'sentient beings' that we can find the proper place for our experience. That we are so grandly and vastly outnumbered also reminds us of our place in the larger scheme. By naturalizing our suffering in this way Darwin is not encouraging us to seek it out. It is, Darwin intimates, morally improving not to regard suffering as morally improving. That it is inevitable does not require of us that we should make it a virtue. And this then raises by implication the question of what, if anything, we are to do about it; of what stories we would be better off telling about this ineluctable fact. What would we want a privileged vocabulary about suffering to do for us, now that suffering, without God as its cause, or its judge, has been rescued from its old descriptions?

'Formerly', Darwin continues, 'I was led by feelings ... to the firm conviction of the existence of God, and of the immortality of the soul':

> In my Journal I wrote that whilst standing in the midst of the grandeur of a Brazilian forest, 'it is not possible to give an adequate idea of the higher feelings of wonder, admiration and devotion, which fill and elevate the mind'. I well remember my conviction that there is more in man than the mere breath of his body. But now the grandest scenes would not cause any such convictions and feelings to rise in my mind ... The state of mind which grand scenes formerly excited in me, and which was intimately connected with a belief in God, did not essentially differ from that which is called the sense of sublimity.

What Darwin is celebrating here is the 'wonder, admiration and devotion' evoked by natural scenery without belief in God; without needing a God in order to feel such feelings. Whatever the presumed existence of God had added to these words, his newly discovered absence doesn't seem to deplete them, or indeed nature itself. If there is no more in man than the mere breath in his body – nothing immortal – this might reinforce a sense of the sublimity of nature. The prolific contingency of life might be more awesome than its divine creation (as though we could have great art without an artist, and not worry about it). What was beautiful about nature – apart from its apparently irresistible aesthetic satisfactions – was that it was unsanctioned. It was not designed by a moralist; it was not designed at all. It simply evolved. It was as transient as our brief breath. And if the world was not the product of an intelligence, how then should we assess the products of our own so-called intelligence?

What Darwin refers to as the 'sense of sublimity' is itself an interesting phrase, given that the experience of the sublime was essentially that which was beyond the making of sense: it was about what overawed us. Whatever was in excess of a person's capacity for representation – whatever threatened our belief in our languages – was sublime ('The sublime,' Thomas Weiskel wrote, 'revives as God withdraws from an immediate participation in the experience of men.'). It is the immediate (in the literal sense) participation of nature in the experience of men and women that Darwin is promoting. But it is the ordinary sublime of transience that he singles out; there is nothing more ordinary, more natural, than that we should have experiences that no one, not even a God, understands: experiences that satisfy us because they overwhelm us, experiences we value because they are strange. The death of God is the death of someone knowing who we are. Just as a criminal is someone who needs to find out about the law, a (Darwinian) naturalist is someone who has to find out about God: what believing in God does for us, so that when you take it away the whole experience of believing changes (just as you can only get a picture of a problem by noticing all the things that don't seem to solve it). If God, Darwin intimates, is no longer the object of our love – our wonder, admiration and devotion – then our sense of what love is, or might be, changes. To love God, for example, is to love someone (so to speak) who is in a position to judge us, who holds the keys to the kingdom of morality; nature, as Darwin describes it, can never take up such a position. So Darwin invites us to imagine, among other things, what it would be like to love without being judged in return; to suffer without assuming that our suffering always has moral validity; and so always to be suspicious of the ways in which we are likely to justify the suffering of others and ourselves. Nature, Darwin insists, is not another word for God.

For Freud, as for Darwin, nature was not God – had not even come out from under God's overcoat – because God was essentially immortal and omniscient; and it was fantasies of permanence and of knowledge that psychoanalysis would do so much to undermine. In another beautiful natural setting – not the Brazilian jungle, but the Dolomite mountains – Freud describes a similar, modern situation of justifying a love of nature. In his 1916 paper 'On Transience' he describes a walk through what is unfortunately translated as 'smiling countryside' in the company of a 'young but already famous poet'. Immediately this appropriately brief dialogue, at its most allegorical, is a debate between Art and Science; and it is the poet who reveals a quasi-religious sensibility. 'All that he (the poet) would otherwise have loved and admired seemed to him to be shorn of its worth by the transience which was its doom.' But Freud 'disputes the pessimistic poet's view that the transience of what is beautiful involves any loss in its worth. On the contrary, an increase! Transience value is scarcity value in time. Limitation in the possibility of an enjoyment raises the value of the enjoyment.' Freud, for whom exclamation marks were themselves a rarity, insists that it is impermanence that confers value; it is the fact of death, of the prodigal forms of transience, that creates pleasure. As though the wishful fantasy of everlasting satisfaction was itself, paradoxically, an attack on the possibility of pleasure, a wish to render the experience of pleasure redundant. 'It was incomprehensible, I declared, that the thought of the transience of beauty should interfere with our joy in it.' For Freud we interfere with our joy by wishing it was otherwise. 'The beauty of the human form and face vanish for ever in the course of our own lives, but their evanescence only lends them a fresh charm.' It is life as provisional, and therefore pleasurable, that Freud celebrates. Love at its strongest, Freud implies, is an acknowledgement of transience, not a wilful denial of it. Deaths make life lovable; it is the passing of things that is the source of our happiness. For the young poet, because there is death, because there is transience, there is only tantalization. As though, Freud intimates, there were two kinds of people: those who can enjoy desiring and those who need satisfaction.

It is a question, Freud believes, of our attitude to mourning. For the young poet mourning is deemed to be unbearable; so for him to love what ultimately disappears – unlike God, or eternal Truth – is to torment himself. Because he cannot mourn he cannot afford to love. 'Mourning,' Freud writes, 'so natural to the layman,' is to the psychologist, 'a great riddle, one of those phenomena that cannot themselves be explained, but to which other obscurities can be traced back.' And one of these other obscurities is love. Inability (or unwillingness) to mourn leads to fear of loving, which amounts for Freud to an inability to live. Those in this position, he writes, like people after the war,

> seem ready to make a permanent renunciation because what was precious has proved not to be lasting, [they] are simply in a state of mourning for what is lost. Mourning, as we know, however painful it may be, comes to a spontaneous end. When it has renounced everything that has been lost, then it has consumed itself, and our libido is once more free (in so far as we are still young and active) to replace the lost objects by fresh ones equally or still more precious.

If we can see Freud here hedging some of his bets – we can recover from loss as long as we are young; our substitutes for what we have lost *may* be even better – his intent is nevertheless clear. Refusal to mourn is refusal to live. Mourning is the necessary suffering that makes more life possible. But it does require of us not only an ability to mourn – and since, as Freud says, 'the mind instinctively recoils from anything that is painful', we need our other instincts for life to encourage us – but also the larger capacity to mourn the whole notion of permanence, which we have represented to ourselves as God, or Truth.

But there is also a contradiction here in Freud's reasoning that perhaps accounts for the impasse between himself and the poet. More life is only possible if we can let ourselves mourn; and yet, he says, those who renounce life (and love) are in a perpetual state of mourning. Perhaps those eternal mourners have transferred their allegiance from the permanent to mourning itself. As if they are saying to themselves, as if the young poet believes, that if nothing else lasts, mourning can. This, one could say, is how intransigent the belief in permanence has become through all its traditional reinforcements. The continuity of one's life in a secular world, the reliable surety, could be mourning. Loss not as the acknowledgement that creates pleasure, but as the addiction that kills it. The belief in permanence – the hardest belief to give up – is an attack on pleasure. Good mourning, in Freud's terms, keeps people moving on, keeps them in time; bad mourning becomes something akin to an ascetic personal religion. It is impossible to love life, Freud intimates, without loving transience. Religion shores promises against our ruin. So 'successful' mourning that comes to a 'spontaneous end' is secular. It is, in other words, open-ended, a restoring of appetite. And the open-ended is both Darwin's and Freud's shorthand definition of the new secular world. Appetite moves us by moving on.

The individual person, like the species of which she is a member, is going nowhere discernible (or predictable), and nowhere in particular. But this is not so much a cause of grief as an invitation to go on inventing the future. As Darwin and Freud discover more and more about the powers of the past – about how the present is continually being rushed by the past – they also realize one simple fact: that the past influences everything and dictates nothing. That so-called knowledge of the past neither predicts nor guarantees our knowledge of the future. The future is not caused by the past: it is merely informed by it. And, paradoxically, their new-found finality of death is integral to this open-endedness. The fact that we are going to die says nothing about the future except that we are going to die. Once our death doesn't matter to anyone else but us – not to God, or gods, or nature itself – it matters in a different way. Once there is nothing (or no one) overseeing it, it begins to look different. Darwin and Freud, as we shall see, invent new deaths for us. They have to make our deaths matter in a secular language. And this makes the future, in its turn, a new kind of object of desire.

It is, needless to say, possible to survive and reproduce (and die) without being happy. In other words, Freud introduces more urgently the question of happiness into the Darwinian equation by suggesting that what makes *human* nature a special case is the problem of satisfaction. Between what Darwin takes to be our essential, and therefore natural, need to survive and reproduce Freud places – as a punctuation of the project – our needs for satisfaction. In Darwin's writing people, as animals, may be unhappy, but they are doing what they cannot help but do; in Freud's account people are equally driven, but their unhappiness shows that they are divided against themselves. They always seem to want more than, or something other than, their mere existence and the reproduction of their genetic inheritance. As though our nature is to demand of nature more than it can give. There is always a fantasy life that is a theatre of excess.

For Darwin happiness may or may not accrue from a life, but its aims are clear. The conflicts in a life, inevitable as they are, are unified by the natural purpose of that life. Whereas for Freud a life is also organized around the enigma of its satisfactions. Darwin centres us in nature, and shows us both how and why nature is careless of our pleasure. Freud centres us in nature – the essential nature of what he calls his 'mythology', the life and death instincts – and then shows us how the crucial issue of our happiness throws us into disarray; how our troubled and squandered capacity for satisfaction makes an unconscious life – a life of fraught burials and uncanny retrievals – both necessary and unavoidable. Freud shows us that once you put happiness in the Darwinian picture – once you start taking happiness as seriously as biology, and language as seriously as morality – nature becomes a different kind of problem. We find ourselves asking it questions that only we can answer.

Once happiness matters – and happiness entails the pleasures of justice as inextricable from the pleasures of sexual satisfaction; the possibilities of kindness made sufficiently compatible with a sense of aliveness – so-called biological functions become moral questions.

Darwin reflecting in 1876 on his youthful experiences in the Brazilian jungle, and Freud recounting his conversation with the young poet in the Italian mountains in 1916, are both preoccupied with the traditional question: What are the preconditions for happiness? But this question now comes in a new form: What do we need to believe in order to love nature, and so, by implication, human nature? When Darwin writes about earthworms as gratuitously benign conservers of the earth, and Freud writes against biographers as the often malign and misguided conservers of other people's lives, they start giving themselves the necessary clues to an answer. They do not, though, tell us how to be happy; they tell us (and themselves) what they love and hate.

Darwin Turns the Worm

'O Eve, in evil hour thou didst give ear
To that false Worm, of whomsoever taught
To counterfeit Man's voice...

Milton, *Paradise Lost*, Book IX, 1067–9

Darwin came back, after five years on the *Beagle*, suffering from nature-shock. He was also, of course, suffering from culture-shock. The 'untamed savages' of Tierra del Fuego, the 'villainous banditti-like army' of General Rosas on the Rio Colorado, so much life on board ship with the difficult Captain Fitzroy and the rest of the crew; all of this – and there was much more, as the most cursory reading of Darwin's *Journal* shows – was quite at odds with anything his life before the voyage had led him to expect. And yet it was the sheer drama and diversity and abundance of natural forms, past and present, that was overwhelming. The now legendary number of specimens brought and sent back from the voyage – and that Darwin had to work so hard to place with the appropriate experts – were the most vivid kind of evidence of this almost unmanage-able excess that made classification imperative. After all, what could one do with all this stuff but link it, one way or another, with what was already known? Some-thing had to be done about the extravagance of nature. One could marvel at things being various, at the miracle of creation, as the young Darwin was keen to do; but one also had to count the cost, as Darwin would gradually discover. For Darwin, and his contemporaries, there was a stark question of analogy: What was nature like? And this brought with it – by implication, as it were – one of Darwin's abiding preoccupations: What, if anything, about nature newly conceived (newly analogized) should we now celebrate, or admire, or even, indeed, emulate? After Wordsworth, for example, people could describe in a new way how nature inspired them, what nature could do for them. What Darwin would single out for praise in the natural world after the voyage of the *Beagle* would inevitably smuggle morality back into an apparently heartless, morally indifferent universe.

'The voyage,' Janet Browne writes in her biography,

> had shown him more things than he had ever contemplated at Cambridge, and in ways impossible to conceive beforehand. He knew now that the external world was not the soft green object familiar to English eyes. Strong light and dramatic scenery told an altogether harsher tale, and internal pictures of volcanoes, earthquakes and human beings dancing on the edge of savagery were unforgettable reminders that the earth generally eschewed gentleness.

It was the sublimity of nature – the sheer multiplicity of things, the excess of violent energies – that made the idea of the soft green object look silly, that exposed the terrified cosiness of certain versions of pastoral. 'The weather is quite delicious,' Darwin would write to his wife Emma from Moor Park in 1858, where he had gone to recover, once again, from the turbulence of writing what became the *Origin of Species*:

> Yesterday ... I strolled a little beyond the glade for an hour and a half ... At last I fell fast asleep on the grass, and awoke with a chorus of birds singing around me, and squirrels running up the trees, and some woodpeckers laughing, and it was as pleasant and rural a scene as ever I saw, and I did not care one penny how any of the beasts or birds had been formed.

Nature can be infinitely reassuring, a virtual idyll, if we don't think about its history. The delight, the pastoral, is sustained through the denial of origins. And it was of course his work on species and their origin, and his eventual 'daring and momentous conviction that species were mutable' (in the words of the editors of Vol. 2 of the *Letters*), that would make any satisfaction or consolation we might get from nature morally equivocal. We are always relaxing in the killing-fields.

If beauty is simply the promise of happiness, then it is worth wondering what kind of beauty Darwin found in nature, and what, if anything, it promises. There are well-known – and well-commented-on – visionary moments in the *Origin of Species*. Moments when Darwin's diligent and attentive patience seems to break down, and the text itself begins to aspire to something at odds with its genre: when what George Lewes would call in a review Darwin's 'noble calmness of exposition' turns into a kind of enthusiasm. In the characteristically thorough fourth chapter on Natural Selection, for example, Darwin quite suddenly seems inspired by what threatens to exhaust him:

> Slow though the process of selection may be, if feeble man can do much by his powers of artificial selection, I can see no limit to the amount of change, to the beauty and infinite complexity of the co-adaptations between all organic beings, one with another and with their physical conditions of life, which may be effected in the long course of time by nature's power of selection.

What Darwin values here is clear: the possibility of infinite change, and the aesthetic satisfaction of co-adaptation. He cannot, of course, call it the successful collaboration of species and their environments, but he is describing things working well together. Beauty and complexity are self-evidently good, and they can be found now in the co-adaptation of the ecological system. But it is, I think, this sense of nature's un-limited and often unpredictable variation that most inspires Darwin; and that he returns to in the famous last paragraph of the *Origin*:

> It is interesting to contemplate an entangled bank, clothed with many plants of many kinds, with birds singing on the bushes, with various insects flitting about, and with worms crawling through the damp earth, and to reflect that these elaborately con-structed forms, so different from each other, and dependent on each other in so complex a manner,

have all been produced by laws acting around us. These laws, taken in the largest sense, being Growth with Reproduction; Inheritance, which is almost implied by reproduction; Variability, from the indirect and direct action of the external conditions of life, and from use and disuse; a Ratio of Increase so high as to lead to a Struggle for Life, and as a consequence to Natural Selection, entailing Divergence of Character and the Extinction of less-improved forms. Thus, from the war of nature, from famine and death, the most exalted object which we are capable of conceiving, namely the production of the higher animals, directly follows. There is grandeur in this view of life ... with its several powers, having been originally breathed by the creator into a few forms or into one ...

The passage moves from the traditional pastoral of birds singing in the trees, through a description of the unsettling laws Darwin has discovered, and on to the final, consoling vindication of the pastoral of hierarchy, and the founding Father. If the question of what nature is like has now been answered – it is like a war, in which there is famine and death – there is a reassuring progress myth underpinning it. In this famously bet-hedging conclusion, Darwin suggests this is a justified war, because it produces our most exalted object, the higher animals. And yet, of course, as Darwin well knew, it was precisely this kind of hierarchy, this way of thinking about nature, that his work was questioning. (Twenty years earlier he had written in his journal, 'Man in his arrogance thinks himself a great work, worthy the imposition of a deity, more humble & I believe true to consider him created from animals.') In actuality Darwin was describing a war in which there is no 'great work' or 'exalted object'; it was in no obvious sense a just or an ameliorative war, a war for which there could be any plausible propaganda. This was the bad news Darwin brought to a political ethos committed to progress and economic expansion. 'The problem that spawns (the) confusion within the Darwinian tradition,' Stephen Jay Gould writes, 'may be simply stated as a paradox. The basic theory of natural selection offers no statement about general progress, and supplies no mechanism whereby overall advance might be expected.' 'Darwin's revolution will be completed when we smash the pedestal of arrogance and own the plain implications of evolution for life's nonpredictable nondirectionality.' Nature is astonishingly prolific, but it is a prodigal process going nowhere special, sponsored by destruction and suffering. What is wonderful and inspiring is the possibility of infinite variation and exquisite adaptation; what is daunting and terrible is the cost. Nature is abundant and unremittingly cruel from, as it were, a personal point of view.

The moral dilemma that Darwin can't avoid – and that the movement of his prose tries to manage in these visionary moments in the *Origin* – is: Which side of this equation he offers us – the flourishing abundance or the cruelty – can we allow ourselves, can we afford, to be most impressed by? What are the moral consequences of wanting and valuing what Nietzsche was to call 'more life', whatever the cost? Indeed, given the scale of depredation in the natural world Darwin describes, even if we were to believe in the progress myth, or in a divine sanction for the whole scheme, would the struggle for survival be worth it? Darwin is at once exhilarated and utterly dismayed.

And yet the inevitable moral turbulence in Darwin's writing is soothed by patient enquiry. It is perhaps a comforting irony that Darwin evolved such a genial, collaborative, socially inclusive method of scientific research, to discover the ruthlessness of the natural order. It was no longer clear, in the light of natural selection, the pitiless struggle for survival, the permanent war that sustained life, what there was about nature that we should be inspired by, let alone consoled by. In all this 'bleak uncharitable survivalism', as Desmond and Moore describe it, what is there to celebrate? Well there are, among other things, those 'worms crawling through the damp earth', such an unusual addition to Darwin's more traditionally pastoral list of birds singing and insects flitting. When Darwin writes about earthworms he can only praise them. It is as though, in writing about worms – paradoxically, one could say, given the conventional iconography of worms – Darwin could wholeheartedly protect himself from moral despair. And he could go on writing about morality – about natural history as, among other things, covert moral enquiry about how to live – without recourse to a deity, a progress myth, or an apparently radical politics. It was to be part of Darwin's undogmatic shuffling of the hierarchies to see earthworms – traditionally associated with death and corruption and lowliness – as maintaining the earth, sustaining its fertility. The poor, he would imply, had already inherited the earth: the worms, the poorest creatures of all, Darwin would privilege at the beginning and at the very end of his life as a writing naturalist. 'Never say higher or lower,' Darwin jotted in the margins of a book.

A lifelong enquiry into the origin of species couldn't help but be a lifelong preoccupation with what Darwin referred to as 'morals and metaphysics'. If we put our moral money on variation and survival, opportunism begins to seem more important than kindness. One couldn't be sentimental about earthworms.

Darwin finished revising the diary of his voyage on the *Beagle* in November 1837. And in that same month he – in the concise words of the editors of the second volume of his letters –

> also read the fourth of a series of papers at the Geological Society of London. Three of the papers reported results of his *Beagle* observations. The fourth presented his hypothesis on the formation of mould by earthworms. This explanation of a 'new Geological Power', as William Buckland called it (in his referee's report to the Society of 9 March, 1838), had been developed by Darwin from a suggestion made by his uncle, Josiah Wedgwood II, during one of Darwin's visits to Maer in Staffordshire.

It was someone else's observation – his uncle and future father-in-law's – and it was about his own country. It was of a piece with his *Beagle* preoccupations: another bit of explanation of what we are seeing when we look at the surface of the earth. Why is the earth's surface as it is and what causes it? In Darwin's view, prompted by his uncle, the surface of some of the earth comes from the digestion of worms. Desmond and Moore, as usual, reconstruct the scene with an exemplary vividness. In the garden at Maer,

> Charles now strolled, and Uncle Jos showed him some disused ground where lime and cinders, spread years before, had disappeared into the soil, leaving a layer of loam. Jos assumed that worms had done the work, although he thought such gardening trivia of little consequence to a young man working on a continental scale. Charles disagreed, and from this unprepossessing beginning sprang a lifelong interest in the humble earthworm – a tiny unsung creature which, in its untold millions, transformed the land as the coral polyps did the tropical sea.

Josiah was the source of many good things for Darwin. He provided him with parental approval for his voyage on the *Beagle*, a wife, and an interest in earthworms. And Desmond and Moore are subtle, as ever, in their intimations. These unsung creatures whose untold millions transformed the land enabled Darwin to write, as it were, his version of *The Making of the English Working Class*. Darwin wanted to tell the story of this marginalized, indeed buried, mass of creatures; and he wanted to tell it in terms of their labour. And their labour was a prodigious work of digestion.

Darwin himself, of course, had an amazing amount of material to digest, and that was to change the face of the earth. And, as everyone who is interested in Darwin knows, he was plagued all his life by digestive problems ('My stomach', he wrote to Fitzroy on 20 February, 1840, 'as usual has been my enemy.' Throughout the life and letters one could quote many such remarks). When it came to earthworms, suffice it to say, their digestion worked. Indeed digestion was their work, and it had the most remarkable consequences. Work and digestion – and the links between them – were to dominate Darwin's life. For the idea of work as digestion, and digestion as the body's forced and unforced labour, Darwin turned to the worms.

The four papers read to the Geological Society of London in 1837 are very specific in their focus. Whether Darwin is reporting on 'recent elevation on the coast of Chili', or the 'Deposits Containing Extinct Mammalia in the Neighborhood of the Plata', or about coral formation, or indeed about worms, each of the brief papers reconstructs a hidden drama from the available evidence: a drama in which, as he puts it, 'a change effected imperceptibly is now in progress'. What Darwin is just beginning to need to explain is the relationship between conservation and transformation. As though nature is torn between preservation and effacement. 'The ancient rivers,' he writes, 'like those of the present day, carried down the carcases of land animals, which thus became entombed in the accumulating sediment.' 'Certain coral formations,' he writes, 'act as monuments over subsided land.' The anxiety informing all Darwin's detailed observations and conjectures is that everything disappears. As though he is somehow relieved that the past can be reconstructed at all: that there is any evidence left of the past, of what might have happened. The tombs and monuments are like brief stays against extinction, just the moments before invisibility sets in. What the resilience and abundance of life-forms and fossils suggested, paradoxically, to Darwin, was how sheerly provisional life was. The theory Darwin proposed in his talk on coral formation,

> to include every kind of structure, is simply that as the land with the attached reefs subsides very gradually from the action of subterranean causes, the coral building polypi soon again raise their solid masses to the level of the water; but not so with the land; each inch lost is irreclaimably gone: – as the whole gradually sinks, the water gains foot by foot on the shore, till the last and highest peak is finally submerged.

Even in these very early writings the painstaking, lucid prose of empirical observation breaks into a covert moral and therefore literary dilemma. If nature is described like this, is the genre elegy – mourning and terror for what is 'irreclaimably lost': for what 'gradually sinks' and is 'finally submerged' – or is it the paean of praise for the 'coral building polypi', or indeed, for the 'subterranean forces'? Which is the more impressive, and why might we think so? And what kind of creatures are we – what is human nature like? – if we are inspired by the survivors who flourish? If we go with the coral, so to speak, we still can't ignore each inch of land 'irreclaimably gone'.

It has been part of the legacy of Darwin to make us wonder what claims we can make for ourselves in the light of what has irreclaimably gone. The fossil record itself is paradoxical: by its very survival it hints at what has been irretrievably lost. Darwin, in other words, at the very beginning of his writing life, in these four papers that famously include in the paper on coral formation his 'first published hint of his belief in evolution', is undergoing a muffled spiritual crisis. His own brand of empirical observation pushes him towards a scandalous question, a question both politically and theologically divisive. A question, of course, that he never asks outright: How should we live if we take unredeemable transience seriously? And it is to worms that he turns for what might once have been called spiritual nourishment: for consolation, for inspiration, and even for the joy that for Wordsworth was nature's greatest boon.

'The formation of the superficial layer of earth, commonly called vegetable mould,' Darwin begins his paper 'On the Formation of Mould', 'offers some difficulties in being fully understood, which apparently have been overlooked.' The difficulties have been overlooked because they cannot be seen (and Darwin exploits the pun in 'overlooking': too much looking makes you blind). Darwin, like Freud, always regards what he can see – in this case, the literally superficial layer of earth – as the result of a hidden process. And this process needs to be reconstructed from further evidence. The ground is as it is because something is happening underground; what is visible is, as it were, the end of a story. And this particular story, with its metaphysically suggestive language – the formation of the superficial, the need to look deeper down etc. – begins with worms. And the result of Darwin's simple, brief enquiry will necessitate a change of language. 'From the prevailing use of the expression "vegetable mould",' Darwin writes, 'it would appear that its origin is generally attributed to some effect of vegetation;' but 'the term "animal mould" would in some respects be more appropriate than that of "vegetable mould",' he concludes. Through our overlooking we have mistaken an origin. When it comes to the surface of certain bits of earth, we have been using the wrong language about beginnings. The buried joke in this modest, brief early paper is that worms created the earth. Darwin wants to justify the ways of worms to Man. And it is in the language of amazement and disbelief – a kind of unmock awe – that he frames his argument. First he makes his empirical enquiries, investigations, experiments in recognizably sensible and serious prose; and then the tone changes as he celebrates his improbable proof.

As with the previous three papers in the 1837 series, what Darwin sets out to explain here is a serious disappearance; not of a land mass, or a group of fossilized creatures, but something more commonplace. And the situation is notably one of gain rather than loss. A few years previously, as Mr Wedgwood pointed out, several fields had been covered with lime, or burnt marl and cinders. And yet now, 'These substances, in every case, were buried some inches under the turf.' In one field the cinders had been buried 'about three inches deep'. In one piece of land that was 'waste land fifteen years ago', which had then been drained, ploughed, harrowed and covered with marl, you could now find, 'beneath a layer nearly four inches thick, composed of fine particles of earth mixed with decaying vegetable matter, those substances which had been spread on the surface fifteen years ago'. This land now was a 'tolerably good rather coarse pasture'; so some kind of natural burial was going on, in the service of improving the soil, a natural process akin to ploughing that turns things over. But in this case although, as Darwin notes, 'it may appear trivial at first', it is the worms that do the turning. Indeed it is worm burial that accounts for something Darwin has 'repeatedly observed': 'fragments of pottery and bones buried beneath the turf, in fields near towns'. Worm burial preserves and restores; and the 'whole operation', Darwin writes with marked certainty – 'The explanation of these facts ... I have not the least doubt is the correct one' – is 'due to the digestive process of the common earthworm'.

Worms, en masse, are akin to geologists; 'worms, in their excavations, swallow earthly matter, and ...

having separated the portion which serves for their nutriment, they eject at the mouth of their burrows, the remainder.' Because they cannot swallow 'coarse particles', like lime or indeed pottery and bones, the finer earth they eject begins to cover the surface. Although it may appear 'trivial at first', the 'supposition', Darwin stresses, 'is not imaginary'. Worms collaborate, through their digestive 'work', with Man's attempts to manure and so fertilize his land; hard to believe, but true. 'Although the conclusion may appear at first startling,' Darwin writes at his most persuaded and most persuasive, 'it will be difficult to deny the probability that every particle of earth forming the bed from which the turf in old pasture land springs, has passed through the intestines of worms.' Darwin, of course, was to come to other more startling conclusions, over the next twenty years, that it would be difficult to deny the probability of. But worms in this paper were aiding and abetting the work of Man; and this could be discovered and verified by anybody who cared to look. The worms all working together, as it were, doing an incredible job, 'at a very slow rate, to a much greater depth'. Darwin wants to warn us away from first impressions towards second thoughts: 'Nor, I repeat, is the agency so trivial as at first it might be thought: the great number of earthworms, as everyone must be aware who has ever dug in a grass field, making up for the insignificant quantity of the work each performs.' This has some of the fervent enthusiasm of someone who has discovered an exemplary new tribe; even as it has obvious parallels with the collaborative scientific movement of which Darwin was a part, and which Huxley was to champion.

In this paper, unlike the previous ones, Darwin makes explicit comparison between the animals and Man; in this mundane revelation – which has parodic as well as theological implications – Man is a poor imitation of a worm. In his characteristically modest way Darwin is shuffling the traditional hierarchies; not cutting men down to size, like an arrogant deity, but trying to get them the right size. 'I may conclude by remarking,' he *does* conclude by remarking, 'that the agriculturalist in ploughing the ground follows a method strictly natural; he only imitates in a rude manner, without being able either to bury the pebbles or to sift the fine from the coarse earth, the work which nature is daily performing by the agency of the earthworm.' Art imitates nature, but poorly: in this understated but ironic version of pastoral, Man the agriculturalist is 'rude': uncultivated, uneducated ... uncultured, unrefined, unsophisticated, uncivilized, primitive, ill-mannered, impolite, indecent, dirty, unkind – all nineteenth-century meanings of the word cited by the OED. In this new vision the last will indeed be first; Man is the primitive. In his exhilaration about the worms Darwin adds a Note to the original paper thirteen days after it was delivered, to the effect that worms had been found to be even more competent than originally thought. Having shown in the paper that 'in a field lately reclaimed from being wasteland, three inches of mould had been prepared by the worms in the course of fifteen years ... we now find' that in less than eight years worms have covered the marl 'with a bed of earth of an average thickness of no less than twelve or thirteen inches'. The worms are making their fertile beds at an incredible rate; preparing the ground.

Darwin is not quite saying in this paper, in some comically glib way, that we should aspire to be like worms; though he is saying, in a quasi-Wordsworthian way, that we can perhaps learn something from nature, and especially by noticing and so valuing those at the bottom of the hierarchy: that sophistication, or culture, has more than one meaning and can be found in the oddest places. But what Darwin is certainly saying, by way of consolation and inspiration, is that what is already here works very well. The sublime destructiveness of nature, of which there is no mention in this paper on worms, is matched by something else; something exemplified by the heroic ordinary labour of worms. After the popular scandal of the *Origin of Species* – with its prolific consequences – Darwin would return, at the end of his life, in his last book, to these worms and their cultured (and cultivating) digestion. After the extraordinary work of discovery of his own life, and the desolating losses and burials it would include – of his own mother when he was eight, of three of his children, including his favourite daughter Annie, of family and friends and colleagues – it was to worms he would turn again to restore, I think, a kind of faith; as a valediction. But even in this early paper Darwin had been able to describe, through the worms, that the earth could look after itself; that there were nourishing processes going on beneath the surface. And that nature could also collaborate with what was then called Man, in his efforts to sustain himself. We are more like worms than we might think, and this need not cause us shame (though it may cause us what Freud called 'the laughter of unease'). Between this 1837 paper, 'On the Formation of Mould', and Darwin's final book of 1881, in which the unsung heroes make it into the title, the *Formation of Vegetable Mould through the Action of Worms*, he would find again and again that the sense in which we are in nature, makes the word 'in' redundant. There was a continuum now where once there had only been a discreet, theological hierarchy.

Nature was abundant, but grace was not abounding. A new secular religion of mourning threatened to replace the redemptive futures of traditional Christianity. 'What an enormous field of undesigned variability,' Darwin could proclaim in a letter of 1861. And yet now there was a quite different nuance to what Tennyson had called, in 'In Memoriam', 'regret for buried time'.

Darwin, Desmond and Moore suggest, returned to his interest in earthworms at the point in his life when he was exhausted by the seemingly endless theological controversy prompted first by the *Origin of Species*, and then spurred on by *The Descent of Man*. 'Darwin had reached an impasse,' they write, in the 1870s:

> Religious controversy had deflated him and he hated it. Ten years and he was running out of

answers, tired of repeating himself. After the last revision to the *Origin*, what more was there to say? The world knew all that was worth knowing about his views ... While Mivart [one of his most insistent Catholic critics] worried over the highest member of creation, Darwin worked at the lowest, the worm. With 'the little strength left to me', he was turning to uncontentious subjects.

And yet Darwin's work had made nature an unavoidably contentious subject; natural history writing had lost its innocence. There were no pastoral retreats now, no plausible refuges from the struggle: war is our continuity. But there were ways of writing that could be, so to speak, war by other means. Darwin's own struggle for survival – both intellectual and physical survival – had depleted him; but he still had an appetite for experimentation and writing, and also for writing experiments.

At around the same time that he returns to his earthworms he writes a letter to his son George about writing. George had wanted to write an attack for *The Contemporary Review* on 'future rewards and punishments', theological subjects which, one way and another, had preoccupied Darwin for most of his adult life. Darwin reminds George of Voltaire, who had found that 'direct attacks on Christianity ... produce little permanent effect'; and that 'good seems only to follow from slow & silent side attacks'. Darwin is proposing here a subtle process of erosion, slow and silent like the worms, side attacks not stark confrontation. One might be more effectively polemical by writing about earthworms – and more interestingly ambiguous in one's intent – than by writing about the origin and purpose of life: Huxley's abrupt, rhetorical terrorism wasn't the only way, nor always productive of the most good. Darwin celebrated and supported Huxley's vigorous straightforwardness; but he preferred for himself and his son something more oblique. 'Though I am a strong advocate for free thought on all subjects,' he wrote in 1880,

> yet it appears to me (whether rightly or wrongly) that direct arguments against Christianity and theism produce hardly any effect on the public; & freedom of thought is best promoted by the gradual illumination of men's minds, which follows from the advance of science. It has, therefore, been always my object to avoid writing on religion, & I have confined myself to science.

This letter is itself at once an implicit critique of the language of politics – that it is too explicit to work – and an admission that for Darwin the best way of writing about theology was to write about science. It is not 'direct argument', Darwin argues, that works, but rather the 'gradual illumination of men's minds' produced by science. Conversion experiences, in other words, do not lead to freedom of thought. It is a puzzling form of persuasion that Darwin is advocating: a combination of indirect argument and the gradual accumulation of knowledge provided, over time, by scientific experiment. A rhetorical art married to a scientific method. And Darwin's artful science is nowhere better represented than in his last book, the *Formation of Vegetable Mould through the Action of Worms, with Observations on their Habits*. A book full of scientific experiment and method; but also full of indirect argument, and 'slow and silent side attacks'. But what could there be to persuade people of in a book on earthworms; or, indeed, what could there be to attack?

To begin to answer these questions we have to infer what Darwin is attacking by noting what he celebrates about the worms; and we have to take seriously, but not earnestly, just what it is about earthworms that attracts his careful attention. Darwin constructs his moral universe firstly by choosing – consciously or unconsciously – what interests him about the worms; and then by what he finds to praise them for. After his life's work the moral question has become starker: Is there anything about nature – and so now, by implication, human nature – that can make us feel better? And what kind of better is possible now if nature has no theological sanction, and is unavailable for wishful idealization? Perhaps it is not strange that as Darwin gets so close to his own death he starts writing about worms. And yet what is striking about this last book is that, though it is obsessed by burial, it is, as it were, counter-elegaic. It celebrates the inexhaustible work that makes the earth fertile. And it commemorates, and rejoices in, the powers of digestion. Indeed, it proposes what might be called a secular after-life: the life of the world that continues after one's own death. The battle, the struggle, the war of life are omitted in this book; it is the sheer resilience and inventiveness of nature – 'how strong worms are' and 'the earth which they so largely consume' – that Darwin wants largely to emphasize at the end of his life. And a kind of collaborative generosity, as though worms, contrary to proverbial wisdom, are on the side of life. 'Archaeologists', Darwin writes, 'ought to be grateful to worms, as they protect and preserve, for an indefinitely long period every object, not liable to decay, which is dropped on the surface of the land, by burying it beneath their castings.' And worms also 'prepare the ground in an excellent manner for the growth of fibrous-rooted plants and for seedlings of all kinds'. They preserve the past, and create the conditions for future growth. No deity is required for these reassuring continuities. It is worms that keep the earth abundant; and, indeed, hospitable to people's needs: the need to conserve and thereby reconstruct the past, as Darwin had done in a unique way; and the need for food. Food and history: what else is there? Darwin's worms carried the virtues he wanted to promote, or to rescue from the moral havoc, the ferocious controversy, his work had provoked. Worms were not a refuge; they were a further defence of his position. They buried to renew: they digested to restore.

Worms worked incessantly; but from their point of view, so to speak, they were merely digesting their food in order to survive and reproduce. And this happened to be contingently beneficial, to archaeologists and to seedlings. They were inadvertently generous; not designed for altruism. Not intentionally collaborative; but the way they struggled for survival had spin-offs for other parts of nature. They provided things without meaning to: they were gratuitously virtuous, not determinedly so. Whether or not archaeologists are grateful, the worms will still go on doing what they do. The world is not designed for our benefit and yet it can be, in its own way, contingently hospitable. It is not a miracle that worms are as they are, and do what they do; it is rather, Darwin intimates, our accidental good fortune. Indeed the two things that most move and impress Darwin about earthworms are their astonishing capacity for work, and their sentience. They are by nature – though from Darwin's point of view, in Darwin's description – thoroughly diligent and improbably intelligent. If they were people we might say that they believed in something; that they were committed. 'Knowing what great muscular powers worms possess', Darwin writes, making them sound like unironized heroes of some lost, classical myth. They are like an unacknowledged elemental force.

So it is of some interest that the final paragraph of the book on earthworms is a kind of reprise to the famous final paragraph of the *Origin*. Once again Darwin invites us to contemplate a natural scene; and once again he will lead us from a beautiful prospect to the hidden powers. But in the *Origin* what the eye can't see is 'the laws acting around us', growth, inheritance, variability, natural selection: the struggle for life, and the war of nature. In the book on earthworms Darwin leaves us with a different story: 'When we behold a wide, turf-covered expanse', he writes,

> we should remember that its smoothness, on which so much of its beauty depends, is mainly due to all the inequalities having been slowly levelled by worms. It is a marvellous reflection that the whole of the superficial mould over any such expanse has passed, and will again pass, every few years through the bodies of worms ... The plough is one of the most ancient and most valuable of man's inventions; but long before he existed the land was in fact regularly ploughed, and still continues to be thus ploughed by earthworms. It may be doubted whether there are many other animals which have played so important a part in the history of the world, as have these lowly organised creatures.

It is as though the earth is reborn again and again, passing through the bodies of worms. Darwin has replaced a creation myth with a secular maintenance myth. This is how the earth maintains itself, as fertile and ongoing. And as always in Darwin's writing, with his preference for the indirect, the 'slow and silent side attack', his language hints at a politics and a theology that the content and context of the work seem to disavow. It is the 'inequalities' that have been levelled by worms. Darwin, of course, knew of the connections between land and inequality; knew who the Levellers were. And if, as Darwin has found, the highest creature in creation, Man, prides himself on something that such lowly organized creatures have always been doing, then there is an intimation that there may be parallels and analogies in the social hierarchy; that those at the bottom can do perfectly well what those at the top claim for themselves. 'Lowly organised creatures' – with all its middle-class fears of unionizing – who have played so important a part in the history of the world is surely, as a description, a side attack on something all too topical.

It would be silly to suggest that Darwin was a closet socialist, but integral to the kind of work he did to suggest that he was capable of diverse and subtle sympathies (what in psychoanalytic language might be called 'split identifications': imagining himself as in some way like apparently mutually exclusive groups of people). It is not that the conclusions arrived at in the *Origin of Species* are here, in the book on earthworms, being in any sense repudiated. The turf-covered expanse he asks us to behold, the beauty of its smoothness, are no less the products of the laws he spent his life trying to understand. But something else is being said about the war of nature, and the 'lowest' of its creatures; something about resilience and beneficial accidents: that it may be more marvellous when the world happens to work for us, than to believe that it was designed to do so.

Darwin is continually surprised in this book by what worms are capable of. What we feared (and hoped) was only going on abroad was actually going on beneath our feet, under our very eyes. 'They are cannibals,' he writes, 'for the two halves of a dead worm placed in two of the pots were dragged into the burrows and gnawed.' Their voraciousness – 'how greedily worms devour fat' – is astonishing. And yet at the same time these worms are immensely talented and competent. Clearly these 'lowly organised creatures' have been consistently underrated; they are far more complex than anybody has bothered to notice. 'It is surprising that an animal so low in the scale,' he writes at one point, 'should have the capacity for acting in this manner, as many higher animals have no such capacity.' He is writing about the worms' capacity to use objects to plug up their burrows. But one way or another the lowly, Darwin insists in this book, are underestimated; whether it be ordinary mortals as compared with a supreme deity, or those at the bottom of the social hierarchy. Something, or someone, is not being given sufficient credit. And Darwin perhaps intimates that our political and theological hierarchies themselves – that always double for each other – are just another powerful weapon in the war of nature. In late-Victorian society there was a chronic underestimation of its 'lowest' members: a sense that what was going on underground was at once shocking and dramatically impressive (at its most literal, histories of mining in this period bear this out).

Darwin, in other words, leaves us with a bafflingly simple question the resonance of which he characteristically understates: What would our lives be like if we took earthworms seriously, took the ground under our feet rather than the skies high above our heads, as the place to look, as well, eventually, as the place to be? It is as though we have been pointed in the wrong direction.

Amid much extensive collaboration with his sons, various farmers, corresponding naturalists in India, and so on, the only person in the book Darwin reports having difficulty in convincing about the grandeur of worms – and indeed makes a point of telling us about over several pages – is a Reverend Joyce. Investigating with his son William the capacity of worms to 'undermine' walls, Darwin discovers a significantly 'broken wall' among the ruins of the small Roman town of Silchester, in Hampshire. 'Recently,' he reports, 'excavations have been undertaken by the Duke of Wellington, under the superintendence of the late Rev. J. G. Joyce.' An aristocrat's interest in Britain's Roman past superintended by a clergyman is, for Darwin, invaluable for his interest in worms. The Rev. Joyce, Darwin tells us, is meticulous in recording the excavations as they progress, making 'careful coloured sections', and 'measuring the thickness of each bed of rubbish' ('bed of rubbish' being a particularly evocative phrase in the circumstances). The worms, Darwin firmly believes, have been instrumental in both the breaking down and the burial of the Roman walls and buildings. 'Mr Joyce was at first sceptical about the amount of work which I attributed to worms':

> but he ends his notes with reference to the last
> mentioned wall by saying, 'This case caused me

more surprise and brought more conviction to me than any other. I should have said, and did say, that it was quite impossible such a wall could have been penetrated by earth-worms' ... the sinking [of the Roman pavements, Darwin goes on several pages later] must, as it appears to me, be attributed in chief part to the pavement having been undermined by worms, which we know are still at work. Even Mr Joyce at last admitted that this could not have failed to have produced a considerable effect.

The Romans are no longer at work: Rev. Joyce, Darwin informs us, has died; and it is increasingly less clear in the 1880s what work, if any, the clergy and the aristocracy actually do. But the worms, as 'we know, are still at work'. Rev. Joyce, it is noticeable in Darwin's carefully worded account, doesn't give the worms as much credit as Darwin does.

In this set piece of mild but emblematic controversy, Darwin is never hell-bent on converting the clergy; he just goes on, genially collecting his evidence. He doesn't claim a victory, but he gets an acknowledgement: 'Even Mr. Joyce at last admitted that this could not have failed to have produced a considerable effect.' And the effect, simply by association with the names of the Romans and the Duke of Wellington is to remind us of imperial ambitions, of grandiose projects as against the unambition of the worms.

It is the paradoxical combination of undermining and conserving – as though, when it comes to worms, the conservation is in the undermining, although neither thing is the worm's intention – that fires Darwin's speculative imagination; and that is, indeed, a description of his own work, in its effect if not in its intention. Like Freud, Darwin is interested in how destruction conserves life; and in the kind of life destruction makes possible.

The Death of Freud

... the thought of death is a good dancing partner.
Kierkegaard, *Philosophical Fragments*

In what Freud referred to as a 'bad, barren month' he wrote to his fiancée, Martha Bernays, in 1885, describing his only achievement in what was clearly a desultory time. He was a struggling young doctor of twenty-nine in Vienna, with seventeen minor publications to his name, none of which he would be likely to be remembered for; none of which would be of much interest but for his subsequent writings that made him the Freud we know. The only thing he clearly relishes telling his much missed fiancée is what he would teach us to refer to as a symptomatic act, an acting out of something, a showing of something that he was unable to tell. And it is an act, presumably, that only an unusually ambitious man would perform. 'One intention, as a matter of fact, I have almost finished carrying out,' he writes,

> an intention which a number of as yet unborn and unfortunate people will one day resent. Since you won't guess what kind of people I am referring to, I will tell you at once: they are my biographers. I have destroyed all my notes of the past fourteen years, as well as letters, scientific excerpts and the manuscripts of my papers. As for letters, only those from

the family have been spared. Yours, my darling, were never in danger. In doing so all old friendships and relationships presented themselves once again and then silently received the coup de grâce (my imagination is still living in Russian history); all my thoughts and feelings about the world in general and about myself in particular have been found unworthy of further existence. They will now have to be thought all over again, and I certainly had accumulated some scribbling. But that stuff settles round me like sand-drifts round the Sphinx; soon nothing but my nostrils would have been visible above the paper; I couldn't have matured or died without worrying about who would get hold of those old papers. Everything, moreover, that lies beyond the great turning point in my life, beyond our love and my choice of profession, died long ago and must not be deprived of a worthy funeral. As for the biographers, let them worry, we have no desire to make it too easy for them. Each one of them will be right in his opinion of 'The Development of the Hero', and I am already looking forward to seeing them go astray.

At this point in his life – a crisis he is keen to be blithe about – Freud clearly wants to be the Sphinx, rather than Oedipus who solved its riddle. By getting rid of the written evidence of the past he has unburied that Sphinx again, recovered the riddle of himself, at least for posterity. His past writings – except that writing that connects him with his family and his fiancée – are

'unworthy of future existence'. And this is not exactly
so that Freud can make a fresh start, but so that he
won't have to worry about his prospective biographers
using it all. (That worry could get in his way.) And it is
not the ordinary fame of a posthumous biography that
Freud is looking forward to, but the exceptional fame
of someone who is the subject of a biography *while he is
still alive.* 'I am already looking forward to seeing them
go astray,' he writes, already anticipating the pleasure
of making them suffer. Because they will never have
these writings, his biographers can only go astray, like
a troop of failed Oedipuses. Only Freud will know the
truth about himself, and he will keep his secret (he
notably doesn't consider the possibility that he might
want to read this stuff himself in the future). He
selectively destroys his past to taunt his imaginary
biographers, 'as yet unborn' and going to be unfortu-
nate and resentful people, given what an object of their
desire he will turn out to be. If there is one glaring wish
here it is Freud's wish to become the kind of man
biographers will compete for. But he wants the right
biography to be written, which will only be wrong – or
at least wildly conjectural – because he has destroyed
the crucial evidence. Freud will be getting two pleasures for the price of one: the pleasure of reading his
biographies (in the plural), and the pleasure of watch-
ing, or just secretly knowing that his biographers have
gone astray. He will be a famous riddle, an enigmatic
hero, unsolvable. Freud then wanted to be both the
riddle *and* the Sphinx, which is, one might say, really
having it both ways. The precursor of the Oedipus

complex for Freud was the Sphinx complex: wanting
to be the mysterious monster that asks the impossible
questions; wanting to be an enigma and a challenge to
others. Wishing to understand other people; helping
people to understand themselves, which appeared to
be Freud's professional project; being, that is to say, a
psychoanalyst, was to be a professional Sphinx: the
one who asks, but never answers, the question. Paradoxically, what Freud wanted to protect was the idea
of a person as an enigma, a riddle that one 'solves' at
an absurd, indeed tragic, cost to oneself.

Freud, he writes, 'couldn't have matured or died
without worrying about who would get hold of those
old papers'. It would have been intolerable to die in
the way he obviously wished to die, without the
reassurance that he had had final control of the
interpretation of his earliest papers, by destroying
them. Freud assumes two things: firstly, he wants to
die having secured certain assurances for himself; and
secondly, he assumes that the absence of documen-
tary evidence will lead to more distortion of his life
story, rather than less. As though, if his biographers
had everything, they might get it right. As though he
would have been found out. Destroying his papers
suggests that Freud believed in the truth – or at least
in the possible accuracy – of biographers. There is the
wish not to be known, and the wish to die knowing
that he wasn't known. It is himself as a (classical)
mystery, himself as someone who must keep his own
secrets about the past, that he wants his fiancée to
know about. He wants her to see him as someone

who covers his tracks, but is fascinating, and eventually to be famous.

It is part of our own life story to try and keep control of the stories people tell about us (there is always the story of the stories I don't want people, including myself, to tell about myself). Freud, in this letter, already looking at his life from the point of view of his impending death, did not want people to know how he had become not only who he was, but who he would become. He had destroyed the tangible traces of his early writing. For his future biographers Freud's writing life will start when he is twenty-nine. And yet, of course, the profession Freud was to invent, and that *would* make him famous, organized itself around two fundamental questions: How do people become who they are? and: What constitutes evidence for this (psychoanalysts, for example, unlike biographers, don't tend to use written documentation, only people's hearsay about themselves)?

Freud was to suggest that the ways in which we tried to destroy our lives (and our life stories) were integral to our life stories. That we were always, as it were, tampering with the evidence of ourselves. Indeed, it was the function of what he would later call the death instinct to make narrative coherence impossible; to spoil our life stories and put a stop to them. To spoil the connections we, or other people, might wish to make. 'The death instinct or destructive force,' his daughter Anna wrote, 'serving the opposite aim (from the life instinct) of undoing connections and destroying life.' The death instinct was a mythical force that, by undoing connections and destroying life, also kept lives private. The life instinct was more on the side of the biographer: the death instinct – that 'works silently', Freud would say, in an ominous phrase – kept spoiling the material. The question of biography – of what one person might claim to know about another, on the basis of specific evidence – was linked for Freud with the question of who, or what, decided what a person's real life story was.

Freud's early ambivalence about knowing and being known is essential to the consequent history of psycho-analysis. In his letter to his fiancée he is writing about the pleasure, if not the necessity, of making oneself a mystery to others. As if his own fear about himself might be that he was not sufficiently opaque; and that to be known was to be exploitable: that a fantasy of knowing someone was a precondition of doing what one wanted with them. We see Freud consciously doing here what he was to become so adept at describing: the way we disguise ourselves to secure certain obscure satisfactions, the way we can only reveal ourselves by hiding. After all, by burning his papers Freud is trying to find a form of hiding that will promote seeking (by the end of the nineteenth century, the future biography was part of the total fantasy of being a writer). Freud was clearly interested in how people flirt with being known; but he was, by the same token, wondering whether there was such a thing as an understanding between people. Why we might want to believe that we are intelligible to ourselves and others was what preoccupied Freud from the beginning, and not merely how we could get better and better at doing it. It is as though he is asking, even in this early letter: What is the wish for understanding a wish for? And if understanding isn't our best currency, our most useful project, then what is? If you write your future wife a letter about how you like to ward off people who are interested in you, you are implicitly promoting alternative kinds of pleasure. A life, for example, might become a search for experiments in living, rather than a quest for recognitions. It might be more about finding pleasurable ways of getting on with people than good ways of knowing them.

What Freud was rather luridly to refer to as a death instinct was, among other things, a way of expressing his scepticism about people knowing and being known by each other. So Freud's discovery of trans-ference – our invention of others on the basis of past relationships – should be seen as part of a larger problem. It's not that we misunderstand each other, that we keep getting it wrong, it is that we put so much belief – false belief – in the whole notion of knowing and understanding. The so-called death instinct then represents that part of ourselves that determinedly wishes not to know; the part of our-selves that is sceptical, as it were, about our belief in knowledge and truth. Freud's wish to make his death instinct unequivocally 'bad' (and his life instinct 'good') obscured the sense in which it carried for Freud some of his more troubling values, rather as Milton's Satan did for Milton in *Paradise Lost*. The death instinct, one might say, was not on the side of the kind of life the life instincts were supposedly on the side of. If we think of these instincts as characters in Freud's drama – as useful fictions but improbable facts – then the death instinct becomes a more interesting figure. It does not, for example, believe that life is an epistomological project in which we strive for better and better knowledge of ourselves and others. Instead it promotes the idea that not knowing things will get us the life we want. The parodist of our truth-seeking, the ironic saboteur of our will to be good, the death instinct becomes the silent unsettler of our lives, and not merely the nihilist lurking in our souls.

So analysing a transference, for example – the defining practice of psychoanalysis as a therapy – may not be a way of making people more realistic in their perceptions of others (the question 'Realistic from whose point of view?' will never go away); but rather of curing them of their belief in their 'knowledge' of themselves and other people. It is not merely that we might be endangered by people's assumed knowledge about us, or our assumed knowledge about them – as in racist and sexist fantasy – but that it is misleading to assume that it is knowledge that we want or that we have of people, any more than it is knowledge we get from listening to music. (Perhaps bodies simply affect each other, or evoke each other.) Biography, for Freud, was a monument to the belief that lives were there to be known and understood, rather than endlessly redescribed. Biography did to the dead what Freud feared psychoanalysis might do to the living.

'What Freud is aiming at', the French psychoanalyst Jean Laplanche writes, 'is a kind of history of the unconscious, or rather of its genesis; a history with discontinuities, in which the moments of burial and resurgence are the most important of all.' This burial and resurgence that one might track – as both Darwin and Freud did in species and in individuals – made the whole notion of the discontinuity of lives neither the problem nor the solution. It was just the nature of a human life to be elusive as an object of knowledge. The idea of a life having a shape, or being a discernibly coherent story, could seem nonsensical. It would be like assuming a life was like a biography; and that the future was something we could look back on.

'If we are to take it as a truth that knows no exceptions,' Freud writes in 1920, in *Beyond the Pleasure Principle*, 'that everything living dies for internal reasons – becomes inorganic once again – then we shall be compelled to say that "the aim of all life is death"...' Everything living is in fact struggling to die. But Freud is not merely saying that living creatures inevitably die; he is suggesting that death is an object of desire. And like all objects of desire – like all Freudian stories about desire – it is something of an obstacle course. But the oddity of this life story that is a death story prompts Freud into some quasi-evolutionary myth-making. What makes life so hard for us all now is that it has become so difficult to die. In fact once life started living the first thing it had to do was find an efficient way of dying:

The attributes of life were at some time evoked in inanimate matter by the action of a force of whose nature we can form no conception. It may perhaps have been a process similar in type to that which caused the development of consciousness in a particular stratum of living matter. The tension which then arose in what had hitherto been an inanimate substance endeavoured to cancel itself out. In this way the first instinct came into being: the instinct to return to the inanimate state. It was still an easy matter at that time for a living substance to die; the course of its life was probably only a brief one, whose direction was determined by the chemical structure of the young life. For a long time perhaps, living substance was thus being constantly created afresh and easily dying, till decisive external influences altered in such a way as to oblige the still surviving substance to diverge ever more widely from its original course of life and to make ever more complicated detours before reaching its aim of death.

Life is a tension which seeks to extinguish itself, to 'cancel itself out'. The first instinct arises, paradoxically, to rid itself of instinct. Something sufficiently vague – 'a force of whose nature we can form no conception' – stirred up some life; and the first response of this new life was to return to its origins, to inanimate matter. But it was better in the old days: 'It was still an easy matter at that time for a living substance to die,' Freud says. There is something unbearable about life – and perhaps by (Freud's) implication, consciousness – some 'tension' that only death can release us from. 'Every man,' Borges wrote, 'runs the risk of being the first immortal.' Every living creature, Freud speculates, is hungry, indeed ravenous for death. But – and this is where the plot thickens – not for any old death. If what Freud calls 'living substance' is prepared to make ever more complicated detours before reaching its aim of death, then it is not any old death it is after. 'We have no longer to reckon,' Freud writes, 'with the organism's puzzling determination (so hard to fit into any context) to maintain its own existence in the face of every obstacle. What we are left with is the fact that *the organism wishes to die only in its own fashion*' (my italics). There is a death, as it were, that is integral to, of a piece with, one's life: a self-fashioned, self-created death.

I think it is worth spelling out just how drastic – and bizarre – Freud's assertion here is. Everything we might have described a life as being about – reproduction, happiness, justice, and of course survival – are all subsumed by this primary project of the organism dying only in its own fashion. We are satisfied, so to speak, only when the wish for satisfaction has disappeared (in death); and yet essential to this satisfaction is that we do it in our own way. 'Hence arises the paradoxical situation that the living organism struggles most energetically against events (dangers, in fact) which might help it to attain its life's aim rapidly – by a kind of short-circuit.' We are, in other words, perfectionists to the end, the artists of our own deaths. Not, of course, conscious artists – the person I recognize myself to be is not plotting this – but inspired by oblivion. The struggle is to have the self-fashioned death.

There are, of course, obvious questions about all this. How do you know – or rather when do you know? – that you are dying in your own way? Isn't this the ultimate omnipotence – projected back into the organism's nature – conceiving of one's death as, ideally, non-contingent, designed by oneself. Isn't this Freud once again seduced back by a spurious, albeit ironized, teleology; one's life does have a project, a purpose, a destiny, a potentially coherent story. 'To die *only* in its own fashion'; as though my death belongs to me; and therefore that someone else, or something else, might take it away from me.

If we are to think of Freud's writing as – among many other things – autobiography-as-theory, auto-biography set to theory, as it were, then we have to ask: What kind of object of desire was death for Freud? What was he writing about when he wrote about death? If there is an idealization of unconsciousness in his growing preoccupation with death – the propo-sal of a death instinct (what Pontalis calls the 'death work') – there is also an abiding enigma about the plotting of lives. By 1920 Freud needed the notion of a death instinct – a curious phrase in itself – to tell more persuasive, more convincing life stories: stories about how people actively, if unwittingly, undo their lives; and how this is a source of satisfaction to them.

An instinct, one might say, is the biological word for

a plot. Something inevitably happens to us when we are born, Freud says, which shapes our lives: we desire. From this point of view the story of our lives is the story of – to borrow one of Freud's titles – our instincts and their vicissitudes (or destinies, as the French translation has it). And yet, Freud asserts in 1920, above all, or rather beneath it all, we desire to die; or rather, to fashion a death. 'Beneath it all,' Larkin writes in his poem 'Wants', 'desire of oblivion runs;' as though oblivion desires us. In Freud's mysterious Ur-creation myth, it is indeed as though life is resistant to itself; oblivion is the subject and the object of desire. For Freud the original life story was a death story, a how-to-die story.

But this cosmic death story is in two acts. First, at no definable moment, and by no describable agent or process, 'The attributes of life were at some time evoked in inanimate matter by the action of a force of whose nature we can form no conception.' The beginning of the whole story, that is to say, defies representation. Life happened to come to life; but the tension this caused was okay because, 'It was still an easy matter at that time for a living substance to die.' Phobic of itself, life could easily get out of itself; it could leave the moment it arrived (get the whole farce over with). And then for equally mysterious reasons – reasons Freud is unwilling or unable to go into – the next thing happened. It is as close as Freud ever gets to describing a version of pastoral, of benign beginnings. 'For a long time, perhaps,' he writes, 'living substance was thus being constantly created afresh and easily dying, till decisive external influences altered in such a way as to oblige the still surviving substance to diverge ever more widely from its original course of life and to make ever more complicated detours before reaching its aim of death.' Something happens of psycho-geological proportions from outside that makes dying more difficult; and that seems to evoke in what Freud calls 'living substance' either a new wish, or the elaboration of an old wish, the wish of the organism to 'die only in its own fashion'. And this new wish is so strong that what Freud calls a 'paradoxical situation' arises. The organism will struggle keenly against dangers that would kill it, 'which might help it to attain its life's aim rapidly,' in order to guarantee the satisfaction of its constitutive wish: to die in its own fashion. And this, Freud remarks knowingly, 'is ... precisely what characterises purely instinctual as contrasted with intelligent efforts'.

In our intelligent behaviour we struggle, rather naively, to survive; but at the level of instinct, at some putatively more profound level, we are also trying to secure our own idiosyncratic death. There is a deep wish not exactly to survive – or indeed do any of the things that culture offers us to legitimate our lives – but to die in our own way. My only project – and it is instinctual, that is to say, unconscious and natural – is my own death. Philosophy, Montaigne famously wrote, following Plato, was about learning how to die; for Freud dying is, by definition, something we do not need to learn. It is not a form of knowledge. Indeed our learning (what Freud calls our 'intelligent efforts') is beside the point. How to die in my own fashion is something that I cannot learn; I might be able to live in my own fashion – by undergoing psycho-analysis, say – but what would be the point?

There are, I think, two questions here that are linked. Firstly, what was the problem the notion of the death instinct was needed in order to solve? In other words, what was Freud hearing in the life stories of his patients – and experiencing in his own life – that only the existence of a death *instinct* could explain? A notion that by his own acknowledgement was excessively speculative ('Since the assumption of the existence of the instinct,' he writes, 'is mainly based on theoretical grounds, we must also admit that it is not entirely proof against theoretical objections'). And secondly, why was Freud so anti-biography – so incensed and baffled, as we shall see, when the writer Arnold Zweig suggested, in 1936, that he write Freud's biography?

Freud needed the odd notion of a death instinct to explain the absolutely obscure apparent purposive-ness of a life in which what looked like self-destructive behaviour was integral to the unconscious logic of that life (and so, of course, could never be amenable to psychoanalysis). People are not, Freud seems to be saying, the saboteurs of their own lives, acting against their own best interests; they are simply dying in their own fashion (to describe someone as self-destructive is to assume a knowledge of what is good for them, an omniscient knowledge of the 'real' logic of their lives).

Biography, in seeming to account for a life, denies the essentially unformulatable logic of a life. A life is a riddle without a Sphinx. It was perhaps inevitable, given how ambivalently committed he was to the therapeutic value of the to and fro between oral autobiography and oral biography that is psychoanalysis, that Freud would not be able to bring himself, at a more immediately personal level, to believe in a biography about himself (how this affected the future biographers he had longed for as a younger man we shall also see). His own *An Autobiographical Study*, published in 1925, could not be more misleadingly titled; it is, more exactly, an autobiographical study of Freud's psychoanalytic movement. Indeed Freud acknowledges this in a Postscript he wrote for an American edition in 1935. 'Two themes run through these pages,' he writes:

> the story of my life, and the history of psychoanalysis. They are intimately interwoven. This Autobiographical Study shows how psychoanalysis came to be the whole content of my life and rightly assumes that no personal experiences of mine are of any interest in comparison to my relations with that science.

Freud, who had invented a new kind of oral autobiography – a life-story therapy – managed to write an autobiographical study with virtually no personal experiences in it. He was not, as we shall see, impressed by the idea of biographical truth. But then, of course, life stories, and the avoidance of life stories, were integral to Freud's work, both clinically and theoretically. The life story was, in part, the ways in which a person avoided having a life story. How we escape from our lives is our life; and how our lives tend to resist our stories about them was what interested Freud.

So perhaps it is worth remembering, in the light of this, Freud's fiction, which I described earlier, about the emergence of life; his fiction of beginnings. The difference between dying as quickly as possible and dying in one's own fashion could also be the difference between having a story to tell – having a life story, even if it's only the story of how one died – and not needing one. Indeed, what is narrative about if it is not about objects of desire and the detours and obstacles and dangers entailed in their acquisition? At a certain point in the dark and distant past, Freud intimates, people began to have life stories. Lives acquired something akin to a narrative structure; there was a new object of desire – not merely death, but dying in one's own fashion – and because it was inevitably an obstacle course, it was like what we think of as a story. And if we lift this poetic fiction out of the mists of fantastic, quasi-evolutionary time, we can also redescribe it by simply saying that there is a part of the self that wants not to have a life story (or to tell it), and there is another part of oneself for whom a life story is inextricable from a life. And so when Freud, in a kind of summation – or at least in a late formulation – of his work, asserted in *Civilization and its Discontents*, in 1930, that 'the phenomena of life could be explained from the concurrent or mutually opposing action of these two instincts ... as well as Eros there was an instinct of death', he was saying that it is as if there are two kinds of life stories going on inside us. From the point of view of the death instinct – that Freud is inclined to regard as the omniscient narrator – my life is a story about dying in my own fashion. From the point of view of the life instinct, of Eros, more life is being sought and sustained. '...Beside the instinct to preserve living substance and to join it into ever larger units (Eros),' Freud writes, 'there must exist another contrary instinct seeking to dissolve those units and to bring them back to their primaeval, inorganic state.'

Freud, of course, like the great poets he admired, is inspiringly inconsistent and muddled. By the time of *Civilization and its Discontents* the emphasis is no longer on the organism dying in its own fashion but more on the death instinct as regressive, aiming to bring life back to its primaeval, inorganic state; in other words, to death. So here it would seem Eros wants to tell stories, more-life-stories, and Thanatos, the death instinct, wants to spoil them, to put a stop to them in its own unique way. To be or not to be is the abiding preoccupation. In 1920 it was a question of dying as soon as possible, or dying in one's own fashion, of having a story; by 1930 there are two stories: the story of how I have tried to put a stop to my having a life story, and the story of how I have gone on having a story to tell; joining my life 'into ever larger units', as Freud says. There is, as it were, my autobiography

84

and my anti-autobiography; and then, perhaps, the biography.

'I am profoundly happy,' Arnold Zweig wrote to Freud in 1936, 'when I see that human life has been put right through your achievement, and in fact that the distortion of human life has become reparable through you. But people understand all this only when it is pointed out to them. That is why I toy constantly with the idea of writing your biography.' Freud replies to this grandiose assessment with an unusually strident counter-claim: 'alarmed by the threat that you,' Freud writes, 'want to become my biographer':

> you, who have so much better and more important things to do, you who can establish monarchs and who can survey the brutal folly of mankind from a lofty vantage point; no, I am far too fond of you to permit such a thing. Anyone who writes a biography is committed to lies, concealments, hypocrisy, flattery and even to hiding his own lack of understanding, for biographical truth does not exist, and if it did we could not use it. Truth is unobtainable, mankind does not deserve it, and in any case is not our Prince Hamlet right when he asks who would escape whipping were he used after his desert?

Freud uses the occasion of his own possible biography to be perhaps surprisingly vituperative about the whole genre; the genre itself, of course, a kind of rival of his own discipline. Both psychoanalysis and biography, after all, cannot help address the questions: What is the truth, if any, of a person's life? are some versions truer than others? and if so, what are the criteria for such judgements? And: what is this truth – or are these truths – for? The whole issue seems to prompt in Freud that kind of dazzling logic he has taught us how to read. 'Truth is unobtainable, mankind does not deserve it, and in any case...'; there is something to protest too much about here. What seems to ruffle Freud is the whole notion of getting at the truth about a person's life; and of the relationship between biographer and subject, prone as it is, he suggests, to 'lies, concealments, hypocrisy, flattery' and the biographer's 'hiding his own lack of understanding' (for biographer here read also psychoanalyst). Lives cannot be got right in the writing – 'truth is unobtainable' – but also (or rather, *and* also), if it was obtainable it would be disillusioning, '...and in any case is not our Prince Hamlet right when he asks who would escape whipping were he used after his desert?' We would all be revealed, that is to say, as punishable, as criminals. Guilty, perhaps, of having lived; of having come to life. Hamlet is brought on, as often in Freud, to tell us the truth about truth.

Actors – people who, like biographers, bring other people to life – are, Hamlet proposes here (Act 2, ii, 511), the best biographers of an age:

HAMLET (to Polonius): ...Good my lord, will you see the players well bestowed? Do you hear, let them be well used, for they are the abstracts and brief chronicles of the time. After your death you were better have a bad epitaph than their ill report while you live.

POLONIUS: My lord, I will use them according to their desert.

HAMLET: God's bodykins man, much better. Use every man after his desert, and who should scape whipping? . . .

If 'every man' was used after his desert, he would be punished. Everybody deserves to be punished: that is why people should not be given what they deserve. The issue here, as in biography and psychoanalysis, is: What are people really like? Freud is quoting Hamlet, who is talking about actors (and Jenkins glosses 'whipping' in the Arden *Hamlet*: 'the statutory punishment for unlicensed players, who were held to be vagabonds'. So Hamlet and Polonius may also be talking about actors who aren't real, legitimate actors). This is, one might say, an infinite fictive regression. And yet, on the other hand, there is something that Freud and Hamlet agree upon, though for different reasons. Everybody is worse than they seem: they present themselves as they would like to be seen, not as they are. The truth is – whatever else may also be true – that people are fundamentally punishable; that they are guilty because they are both criminals and imposters. Whether it be the scar of original sin – 'God's bodykins man' – or the guilt consequent upon their instinctual endowment, or the guilt of duplicity, they deserve to be punished; and they may need to die. Hamlet's suicidal browsing and brooding is, among other things, about how difficult it is to die; or even to die in one's own fashion, according to one's own wish.

There are then, Freud suggests, two true stories – whether or not they can be accurately construed – that constitute the individual's life story: the story of how one dies in one's own fashion, and the story of one's guilt. And Freud in his misgivings about biography – which may also be his displaced misgivings about psychoanalysis itself – insists that both stories are virtually inaccessible to the biographer, if not to the person himself. So Freud's critique of biography is firstly, that it cannot tell us what we most want to know; and secondly, that we can never trust the motives of the biographer ('What does the biographer want?' is analogous to 'What does the analyst want?').

In his speech on receiving the Goethe Prize in 1930, Freud once again raises the question of our relationship with the dead, the mourning that is biography. 'We all,' Freud writes,

> who revere Goethe, put up, without too much protest, with the efforts of his biographers, who try to recreate his life from existing accounts and indications. But what can these biographies achieve for us? Even the best and fullest of them could not answer the two questions which alone seem worth knowing about. It would not throw any light on the

riddle of the miraculous gift that makes an artist, and it could not help us to comprehend any better the value and effect of his works. And yet there is no doubt that such a biography does satisfy a powerful need in us. We feel this very distinctly if the legacy of history unkindly refuses the satisfaction of this need – for example in the case of Shakespeare ... But how can we justify a need of this kind to obtain knowledge of the circumstances of a man's life when his works have become so full of importance to us? People generally say that it is our desire to bring ourselves nearer to such a man in a human way as well. Let us grant this; it is, then, the need to acquire affective relations with such men, to add them to the fathers, teachers, exemplars whom we have known or whose influence we have already experienced, in the expectation that their personalities will be just as fine and admirable as those works of art of theirs which we possess.

It is as though, Freud suggests, biography provides a necessary but suspect, or even spurious, intimacy with the great dead. Freud implies – along the lines of his references to Hamlet for Zweig – that our 'expectation that their personalities will be just as fine and admirable' as their works can only be disappointed. There is a disillusionment to be averted; because the best versions of a person are in their works (and if this is true then one might argue that the connection between their lives and 'personalities' and their work might be *more* rather than less interesting). How does it happen that such a disappointing creature can produce such 'fine and admirable' work? Why, in other words, does Freud assume that we can't bear our 'fathers, teachers, exemplars' to be complicated, to be a mixed bag? It is over the question of biography that Freud's commitment to motives as essentially mixed breaks down. He wants to protect the great from their biographers; and so, oddly, it is the biographer who is scapegoated. 'We may admit,' Freud continues, 'that there is still another motive force at work. The biographer's justification also contains a confession. It is true that the biographer does not want to depose his hero, but he does want to bring him nearer to us. That means, however, reducing the distance that separates him from us: it still tends, in effect, towards degradation.' The biographer's relationship to his subject, Freud intimates, is a heady brew of Oedipal triumph and sibling rivalry. But there is also a knot here that Freud doesn't untangle. Does biography degrade because of the motives of the biographer, or because of the human, all too human life of the great artist? Are lives intrinsically degraded objects, and if so, degraded compared with what? (The translator's choice of the term 'degraded' is of interest here, meaning as it does, degeneration and decomposition, as well as loss of dignity.) 'It is unavoidable,' Freud writes ruefully, 'that if we learn more about a great man's life we shall also hear of occasions on which he has in fact done no better than us, has in fact come near to us as a human being.' But, Freud says, rounding upon himself, we can declare 'the efforts of biography to be legitimate' after all, because of what he calls 'the psychological fatality' of ambivalence. Fundamentally man is the ambivalent animal: both the biographer and the great artist are united in their ambivalence; the war between love and hate is the one universal fact of our nature. As a great leveller it is the one description that does us justice.

Once again it is a puzzling, if not a confounding, speculative itinerary Freud has taken us on in discussing biography. Biography is no good because it doesn't tell us what we want to know: the provenance of the artistic gift, and why the work is valuable. But it's okay because it adds to our repertoire of exemplary figures whom we can emulate and identify with (like minor deities). Biography isn't actually any good, because biographers inevitably degrade their subjects; but it's actually fine – legitimate is Freud's word – because we are all ambivalent anyway and therefore degraded, both the biographer and his subject: all compounded of the same virtues and vices. In biography – and perhaps in psychoanalysis – we can't get at the truth about people; and yet the fundamental truth about people is ambivalence. Our lives are, as it were, the way we fill in the details of our own personal ambivalence as it unfolds over time. 'Instincts and their transformations are at the limit of what is discernible by psychoanalysis,' Freud writes; and these, he implies – which are the essence of a person's life in Freud's view – are even less discernible to the biographer.

It is perhaps unsurprising that Freud was fascinated by biography and its impossibility; he works very hard to persuade us how and why the biographer's art is implausible. If he had been a more nonchalant pluralist or relativist he might have been able to say: There are inevitably many versions of a life – perhaps as many as can be told. Some seem more convincing than others and we could, if we wished, try to establish what it is that makes one life story work better than another. But what Freud actually wants to persuade us to do is be suspicious, above all, about biography; to be wary of the apparent coherence and plausibility of life-plots. The only structural guidelines he is prepared to give us in the mapping of lives is the existence of unconscious instincts; the destinies of which are unavoidably recondite and enigmatic for two reasons. Firstly, instinct can only be in any sense known when it is 'translated' into forms of representation that are themselves disguises (the body becoming language in the process of acculturation); and secondly, a person's instinctual endowment (plot-endowment) is subject to contingency, to accident, to circumstance, to the family one happens to be brought up in. And instinct is most influenceable, most set in its way, in childhood. If instinct provides a kind of coherence of need – a desire narrative of appetite and safety – chance keeps disrupting the proto-patterns of our putative biology.

It is not accidental that in Freud's psychoanalytic biography of Leonardo, he pays his most eloquent and insistent tribute to chance; and not simply, or solely, as he does everywhere else, to the daemonic power of instinct. Instinct rushes into an unruly world to be shaped and reshaped. 'If one considers chance to be unworthy of determining our fate,' Freud concludes his 1910 book *Leonardo da Vinci and a Memory of his Childhood*,

> it is simply a relapse into the pious view of the universe which Leonardo himself was on the way to overcoming when he wrote that the sun does not move. We naturally feel hurt that a just God and a kindly providence do not protect us better from such influences during the most defenceless period of our lives. At the same time we are all too ready to forget that in fact everything to do with our life is chance, from our origin out of the meeting of spermatozoon and ovum onwards ... The apportioning of the determining factors of our life between the 'necessities' of our constitution and the 'chances' of our childhood may still be uncertain in detail; but in general it is no longer possible to doubt the importance precisely of the first years of our childhood.

In our lived lives we enact the impact of chance on our early instinctual life. How could a biographer even begin to reconstruct that, when even a psychoanalyst, with a living subject on his couch almost free-associating, finds it so difficult? The inevitable obscurities of the shaping of childhood desire are another nail in the biographer's coffin.

'There is nowhere,' Lacan writes, 'where man's relationship to himself has been less elucidated, nor where his recognition has needed to rise to a challenge more crucial than the one which resonates in classical thought through the statement of Pascal: "a child is not a man".' Freud answered the question: What is an adult? with an analogy as the answer: An adult is like a child. But then, as one analogy always leads to another, the question became: What is a child like? Of course various people, after Freud himself, were to answer this question – most notably Melanie Klein, Anna Freud, Donald Winnicott and John Bowlby. And yet what Lacan alerts us to is whether the question makes sense. What is a child like? and, How do fantasies of childhood (about childhood) figure in an adult's relationship to himself? were the questions psychoanalysis would investigate. And this involves, Lacan suggests, an account of the *differences* between children and adults. How could a biographer, let alone a psychoanalyst, work out such things from any available documents?

It is an insufficiently acknowledged – insufficiently enjoyed – paradox that the more Freud elaborated psychoanalytic theory the less impressed he was by the knowability of the human subject. The possibility of something, some words, one could legitimately call knowledge about oneself or other people seemed increasingly elusive. Both chance, by definition, and instinct by its very (obscure) nature were unpredictable and indeterminate. Useful sense and meaning could sometimes be made retrospectively, but, as Freud could not help insisting, psychoanalysis offers us nothing by way of predicting our lives; it simply shows us – like Darwin's writing – the power of the contingencies we inhabit: our desire, our childhood and our chances. Biography as the monumentalizing of retrospection becomes for Freud a kind of negative-ideal for psychoanalysis. To talk about biography is to talk about – is to have an easy target for – the impossibility of convincingly plotting lives. But it is also a way of talking about the biographical appetite; the hunger of the biographer, and our hunger as readers, for an intelligible life. What, Freud seems to wonder, is an appetite for biography an appetite for? Biography is fraught with difficulty, perhaps impossibility, Freud insists, but we can't resist it. We want something from biography, and what we want may be more or less disreputable.

As the recent so-called 'Freud wars' show – not to mention the endlessly reiterated death of Freud and psychoanalysis claims – interest in Freud's biography, more knowledge about Freud's own life, have become the source book for both the denigration and the promoting of psychoanalysis. Instead of simply being read by people who are moved by or curious about his writing and ignored by those who aren't impressed, Freud continues to be attacked and defended with un-usual relish. He is endlessly worked on and worked over as though he were a disturbing memory. And currently there are thought to be two ways of settling the issue of psychoanalysis: subjecting its practice and theory to scientific criteria, and researching into Freud's life, as though there must be truths to be found, and truths to be tested. And biography and science – incompatible though they may be – are our contemporary touchstones. Freud's work does, after all, insist that all truths, whatever else they may be, are biographical truths, even if the status of these truths is fraught with uncertainty. But Freud's scepticism about biographical truth was as much a covert scepticism about the possibility of truth as it was a misgiving about biography. What psychoanalysis kept showing Freud, despite his wish to the contrary, was that people were not truth-seeking animals in any simple sense; that the concept of truth was a cover story for rather diverse forms of satisfaction.

It is perhaps worth wondering, given Freud's explicit and well documented antipathy to, and preoccupation with, biography, what a psychoanalyst might be doing then – what a psychoanalyst might want – in writing Freud's biography. At its most minimal, any psycho-analyst who writes a biography of Freud is, as it were, promoting the father by betraying him (the second paragraph of Jones's monumental *Life* of Freud reads, guiltily, 'It is not a book that would have met with Freud's own approval'; and Peter Gay's more con-temporary biography begins with anecdotes about Freud burning his private papers. 'Let the biographers labour and toil,' Gay quotes Freud as writing, 'we won't make it too easy for them.'). The biographers in both cases are more than mindful both of Freud's personal misgivings about himself as a biographical subject, and also of the ways in which Freud's theory, as I have suggested, uniquely problematizes the art of

biography: biographers were to Freud what creation-
ists were to Darwin. How, for example, Freud asked
again and again, does a person's death fit into their
lived life? A question, of course, he would not be able
to answer about himself. Only for the biographer is
death an event in life. So I want to turn to the real death
of Freud, in these two of its most authoritative versions; to see both how Jones and Gay want Freud to
die, and how they connect his death to his life. Or, to
put it another way, if the organism wishes to die in its
own fashion, whatever that means, did Freud?

Freud, as we have seen, was continually putting
obstacles in the path of the biographer; at once insis-
tently dissuading people from writing his own biography, and casting aspersions born of psychoanalytic
experience on the genre itself, and the whole notion
of biographical truth. Paradoxically, from Freud's point
of view, to understand human beings was to understand the impossibility of plausible biography; a life
was made and marred by discontinuity, so there can be
no finalizing descriptions. Psychoanalysis revealed
both the dubious motives for biography, and the
absurdity of its truth claims. In so far as lives have
anything resembling a master-plot it is born of the
relationship – for want of a better word – between
unconscious desire and contingency, their mutual
and continuous interruption of each other. Unconscious desire is described by Freud as having an aim
and a (displaceable) object; contingency or chance has
neither. So in the light of these strictures what, briefly,
do Freud's biographers think that they are doing?

Jones, extraordinarily, decided, in agreement with Freud's family, to write his official life because, as he writes in the Preface, 'Ill-natured people were already at work distorting isolated passages [of Freud's work] with the object of disparaging his character, and this could be rectified only by a still fuller exposition of his inner and outer life.' Clearly, anyone who believes in distortion believes there is a real version there available for distortion. Jones implies with his unusual logic, that when we know more about Freud, interpretation of his work will be truer, freer from distortion. His biography aims, in other words, to regain control over what counts as an acceptable reading of Freud's work (as though a biography was not itself subject to a variety of interpretations). The life would be a corrective. Indeed, he goes on, what changed the family's mind about the need for an official biography 'was the news of the many false stories invented by people who had never known him, which were gradually accumulating into a mendacious legend.' Clearly, in Jones's and the Freud family's view, Freud was wrong: there is something like biographical truth which can be distinguished from mendacious legend. A good biography can at least set limits to the acceptable versions of a life. Getting it right is in the service of preventing other people getting it wrong. It is an exercise in damage-limitation. Perhaps biographical truth *is* unobtainable, but biographical *untruth* about Freud seems to be proliferating. The biography aims to protect Freud – the memory of Freud, his image – from something terribly damaging. Let's call the catastrophe, blandly, anyone's freedom to think whatever they like about Freud. And his death, as constructed by his official biography, will spectacularly confirm Freud's own speculations. Freud will be seen to be a man of his word, consistent – that is, narratively coherent – right to the very end. This is Jones's rather moving account of Freud's last days and hours:

> He found it hardly possible to eat anything. The last book he was able to read was Balzac's *La Peau de chagrin*, on which he commented wryly: 'That is just the book for me. It deals with starvation.' He meant rather the gradual shrinking, the becoming less and less, described so poignantly in the book.
>
> But with all this agony there was never the slightest sign of impatience or irritability. The philosophy of resignation and the acceptance of unalterable reality triumphed throughout.
>
> The cancer ate its way through the cheek to the outside and the septic condition was heightened. The exhaustion was extreme and the misery indescribable. On September 19 I was sent for to say good-bye to him and called him by name as he dozed. He opened his eyes, recognized me and waved his hand, then dropping it with a highly expressive gesture that conveyed a wealth of meaning: greetings, farewell, resignation. It said as plainly as possible 'The rest is silence'. There was no need to exchange a word. In a second he fell asleep again. On September 21 Freud said to his doctor:

'My dear Schur, you remember our first talk. You promised me then you would help me when I could no longer carry on. It is only torture now and it has no longer any sense.' Schur pressed his hand and promised he would give him adequate sedation, and Freud thanked him, adding: 'Tell Anna about our talk.' There was no emotionalism or self-pity, only reality – an impressive and unforgettable scene.

The next morning Schur gave Freud a third of a grain of morphia. For someone at such a point of exhaustion as Freud then was, and so complete a stranger to opiates, that small dose sufficed. He sighed with relief and sank into a peaceful sleep; he was evidently close to the end of his reserves. He died just before midnight the next day, September 23, 1939. His long and arduous life was at an end and his sufferings over. Freud died as he had lived – a realist.

For Jones, Freud's death is as exemplary and heroic as his life, a triumph of Freud's belief in the deity he had himself invented, the reality principle. Two things seem to me to be striking about the scene as Jones describes it: firstly that Freud is seen as a pure culture of the reality principle. And the genre of realism Jones uses the death to celebrate is an uneasy mix of classical heroism and British stiff upper lip. Freud's manners are perfect: 'there was never the slightest sign of impatience or irritability;' he is not, as it were, an hysterical woman at his death, but a man facing his

fate without wish or illusion: 'there was no emotionalism or self-pity, only reality.' Indeed reality is Jones's
insistent word: 'Freud died as he had lived – a realist.'
Freud's theory and practice were of a piece; he was,
Jones implies – flying in the face of all the psychoanalytic evidence – a remarkably consistent, heroically
unified subject. A man in whom adherence to the
reality principle has to all intents and purposes extin-
guished the pleasure principle; a man without an
unconscious. The philosophy of resignation and the
acceptance of unalterable reality triumphed throughout. Freud, the man who mastered his unconscious;
the man who lived and died by his own truth.

And yet Freud's last 'highly expressive gesture' said
to Jones 'as plainly as possible "The rest is silence" '. So
Freud was also Hamlet, and Jones Horatio. Jones both
relegates Freud from a father into a son, and links him
implicitly with someone quite at odds with Jones's
noble stoic. The full irony of Freud's reading Balzac's
La Peau de chagrin seems lost on Jones; as is his reading
of Freud's gesture. Freud asks his doctor Schur to kill
him, and so his last wish is, as it were, terminally
diminishing. But the second thing worthy of note in
Jones's account, is that Freud, in one sense, arranges
his own death; he rather too literally dies in his own
fashion. Above all, in Jones's account, Freud must not
be seen to be at odds with himself. He must not be
anything resembling a divided subject. Hamlet, once
again in psychoanalytic writing, provides a loophole.

So it is of interest that when Gay comes to reconstruct the same scene he refers to Freud's last gesture

to Jones – and indeed says 'Jones read Freud's gesture aright' – but omits the reference to Hamlet. Gay clearly wants to unHamlet his hero. This is Gay's account:

> Freud was very tired now, and it was hard to feed him. But while he suffered greatly and the nights especially were hard he did not get, and did not want, any sedation. He could still read, and his last book was Balzac's mysterious tale of the magical shrinking skin, *La Peau de chagrin*. When he had finished the book he told Schur, casually, that this had been the right book for him to read, dealing as it did with shrinking and starvation. It was the shrinking, Anna Freud thought, that seemed to speak particularly to his condition: his time was running out. He spent the last days in his study downstairs, looking out at the garden. Ernest Jones, hastily summoned by Anna Freud, who thought her father was dying, stopped by on September 19. Freud, Jones remembered, was dozing, as he did so much these days, but when Jones called out '*Herr Professor*,' Freud opened an eye, recognized his visitor, 'and waved his hand, then dropped it with a highly expressive gesture that conveyed a wealth of meaning: greetings, farewell, resignation.' He then relapsed into his doze.
>
> Jones read Freud's gesture aright. Freud was saluting his old ally for the last time. He had resigned from life. Schur was agonized by his inability to relieve Freud's suffering, but two days after Jones's visit, on September 21, as Schur was

sitting by Freud's bedside, Freud took his hand and said to him, 'Schur, you remember our "contract" not to leave me in the lurch when the time had come. Now it is nothing but torture and makes no sense.' Schur indicated that he had not forgotten. Freud gave a sigh of relief, kept his hand for a moment, and said, 'I thank you.' Then, after a slight hesitation, he added, 'Talk it over with Anna, and if she thinks it's right, then make an end of it.' As she had been for years, so at this juncture, Freud's Antigone was first in his thoughts. Anna Freud wanted to postpone the fatal moment, but Schur insisted that to keep Freud going was pointless, and she submitted to the inevitable, as had her father. The time had come; he knew and acted. This was Freud's interpretation of his saying that he had come to England to die in freedom.

Schur was on the point of tears as he witnessed Freud facing death with dignity and without self-pity. He had never seen anyone die like that. On September 21, Schur injected Freud with three centigrams of morphine – the normal dose for sedation was two centigrams – and Freud sank into a peaceful sleep. Schur repeated the injection, when he became restless, and administered a final one the next day, September 22. Freud lapsed into a coma from which he did not awake. He died at three in the morning, September 23, 1939. Nearly four decades earlier, Freud had written to Oskar Pfister wondering what one would do some day, 'when thoughts fail or words will not come?' He could not suppress a 'tremor before this possibility. That is why, with all the resignation before destiny that suits an honest man, I have one wholly secret entreaty: only no invalidism, no paralysis of one's powers through bodily misery. Let us die in harness, as King Macbeth says.' He had seen to it that his secret entreaty would be fulfilled. The old stoic had kept control of his life to the end.

Freud, Gay says, 'had resigned from life'; that is, he had not been sacked from life, he had decided not to do the job any more (he had resigned, he hadn't retired). Despite a life's work committed to the sheer power of unconscious desire, the unruliness of chance, the fragility of the ego; despite a life's work, that is to say, committed to the absurd and tragic helplessness of the individual, his always untimely self-division, 'The old stoic', Gay concludes, 'had kept control of his life to the end.' Freud had done, in other words, what his work had shown to be impossible – to be, in fact, the formative human delusion – that one could keep control of a life. Something, of course, a biography cannot help but try to do. Where Jones's emphasis was on Freud as exemplary realist, Gay's emphasis is on Freud dying in his own fashion, ensuring he has exactly the death he wants, indeed had wanted forty years before. But Gay's excerpt from his letter to Pfister replaces what we might call – for want of a better word – the hedonist in Freud with the stoic. The complete paragraph of the letter Gay quotes reads as follows:

I cannot face with comfort the idea of life without work; work and the free play of the imagination are for me the same thing, I take no pleasure in anything else. That would be a recipe for happiness but for the appalling thought that productivity is entirely dependent on a sensitive disposition. What would one do when ideas failed or words refused to come? It is impossible not to shudder at the thought. Hence, in spite of all the acceptance of fate which is appropriate to an honest man, I have one quite secret prayer: that I may be spared any wasting away and crippling of my ability to work because of physical deterioration. In the words of King Macbeth, Let us die in harness.

This clearly is not Gay's (or Jones's) 'old stoic'; it is the German Romantic writer and usurping murderer, the man who wants to write or die (Macbeth is not Hamlet, nor was meant to be). The biographical truth that both biographers need us to believe is that Freud was, as it were, the master of self-mastery. And above all that he chose his own death, in the full light of its inevitability. He chose, to put it crudely, who would kill him; not impersonal nature, not the Nazis – Freud, as Gay says, 'had come to England to die in freedom' – but his friend and doctor Max Schur. Freud's death was another triumph for medicine.

Freud's work showed the ways in which our lives are at odds with our descriptions of them; indeed, that our descriptions are at odds with themselves. For both Jones and Gay the death, Freud's death, must say something about the life; must prove that the life was discernibly of a piece and that the death, therefore, was of a piece with the life. Freud had come to terms with life, so he is unperturbed by his death. He is notably unfrightened, and he goes gently into it, helped by friends and family. If acceptance of the reality principle means anything it must mean acceptance of death. Freud was, his biographers intimate, at one with his ideas; he embodied his beliefs. He had unified himself.

And yet it was part of the Freudian revolution – that of course pre-dated Freud himself – to undermine this particular genre of the heroic ideal; consistency, coherence, integrity in Freud's redescription of them begin to look complicit with everything that undoes them. Biography, I think Freud believed, could not include the complexities of a life that his work had revealed; in fact psychoanalysis itself struggled to contain its discoveries. Freud's candidates for the making of a life – unconscious desire, the life and death instincts, infantile sexuality, the unconscious, language, primal helplessness, family relationships, chance – do not lend themselves to straightforward intelligibility. To describe a person's life, in Freud's view, is to be describing all this.

But why not? It is, after all, what psychoanalysis does, and what we all do all the time in different ways. We can never say everything, but we can say some things of interest. It is as though, having given us so many novel ways of making sense of our lives, Freud turns against his own creation, in wrathful scepticism. Biography, in all its fixity and formulations – with all its indelibly written evidence – was like a picture for Freud of what psychoanalysis at its worst might become: the patient 'cured' by psychoanalysis believing he was both the author and the subject of his own biography. Biographical truth sponsored the illusion that there could be such truth about a life; indeed it might encourage people to live their lives not for their God, as they once did, but for their biographers. Whereas what Freud hoped were the more truthful truths revealed in a psychoanalysis were nomadic and provisional, spoken and therefore evanescent; subject to the vagaries of internal memory, inciting and resisting revision.

Freud hated biography because it represented the dangerous and misleading claims one person might make about knowing another person. A biography might be like a parodic monument of our wishful relationship to the dead, and to the living. This, Freud seems to say, is what the illusion of knowing another person can turn into; this is what our craving for access to others, especially in their absence, looks like. And the problem for Freud is not merely that an unacceptable or disparaging or idealized version of the subject will be produced, but that biography implicitly claims that biography is possible; that lives can be, in some sense, finalized in our accounts of them. That what biographers do to their subjects is what we are always trying to do to ourselves: agree about who we are. The Freudian word for the biographer is the ego.

Freud wants us to be self-defining creatures, but

self-defining at one remove; not merely the inventions of our conscious will. So he calls the self-defining self 'unconscious desire', partly to show us the ironic sense in which we are the unnameable authors of our own lives (authors who keep losing the plot, authors who experience themselves as being fed their lines from some odd place). And his heroic image of self-defini-tion, of self-fashioning, is the notion that we want to die in our own way. The subject of a biography always dies in the biographer's own way.

Freud's notion of the death instinct, controversial as it has always been – as (metaphysical) fiction of the most implausible kind, a way of starkly accounting for an apparently intransigent aggressiveness or regressive-ness in so-called human nature – has seemed to many people to be Freud's most aberrant but significant fiction. Wilde thought that when people were talking about the weather, they were always talking about something else; when Freud was talking about the terrible internal weather he called a death instinct, he was talking about people's natural (unconscious) furtive independence. Freud, Lionel Trilling wrote in his famous lecture, 'Freud and the Crisis of our Culture',

> needed to believe that there was some point at which it was possible to stand beyond the reach of culture. Perhaps his formulation of the death in-stinct is to be interpreted as the expression of this need. 'Death destroys a man,' says E. M. Forster,

'but the idea of death saves him'. Saves him from what? From the entire submission of himself – of his self to life in culture.

But what, it is also possible to ask, is submitting oneself to culture submitting oneself to, in Trilling's terms? Whatever else it might entail, it entails our submitting ourselves to other people's descriptions; of which biography might seem to be the crudest of examples (every child begins his life being described by his parents). Nature in Trilling's interpretation is a kind of alternative to culture for Freud; as though there are two things in a sado-masochistic relationship, nature forever submitting to culture – bound and whipped and tantalized by it – but asserting its forlorn independence in something called a death instinct. The death instinct as a lease of natural life, a flourish of independence. The death instinct as that part of ourselves that eludes the multiple biographies we submit to – everybody's account of us, including our own – by living in culture.

Thinking about his own biography, which Freud started doing at a young age – and speculating later about the whole nature of biography, its seductions and its reprisals – confronted Freud with the question of his own life after death: his reincarnation in the memories of those who knew him, and the interpretations of those who would read him; and, of course, the bringing together of these things in biography. There was one's own death as an obscure object of desire, and there was the haunting thought of its curious undoing in posthumous fame or notoriety. So many people now would inherit his sentences. What kind of mourning would his death evoke in those who survived him, what would they do, what would he become in people's minds? For Freud – and this is everywhere alive in his nagging obsession with the art of biography – there was an after-life, but not for us. It was the after-life of memory; and it was in this world and not the next. To imagine one's biography – even by trying to stop it being written – is one way of imagining one's own death; like the fantasy of attending one's own funeral, it can only be the ironic wish for more life after life.

The anticipation of our own death tells us more about anticipation than it does about death. Indeed the whole notion of looking forward to something immediately becomes enigmatic in relation to death. The word itself is at once a stark symbol of the future as always opaque, always unknowable; a word without an obvious referent – when one thinks about death one is thinking about life after death, the word itself implying a next stage – it denoted for Freud an object of passionate desire; the lover who ultimately will not refuse us, and yet who takes everyone.

Freud's notion of the death instinct suggests, at its most minimal, that we can want (or need) something we know nothing about, and that we are most drawn to what we think of ourselves as trying to avoid. That we are, essentially, idiosyncratic suicides, but not from despair, but because it is literally our nature to die. But death, in Freud's poetic fiction, is a paradoxical and therefore exemplary object of desire; it is the object of desire that finally releases us from desire. The end, in both senses, of our suffering.

Epilogue

The value of ideals lies in the experiences to which they lead.

John Dewey, *Art as Experience*

For both Darwin and Freud the idea of death saves us from the idea that there is anything to be saved from. If we are not fallen creatures, but simply creatures, we cannot be redeemed. If we are not deluded by the wish for immortality, transience doesn't diminish us. Indeed, the traditional theological conviction that we needed to be saved – the secular equivalent being the belief that we could and should perfect ourselves, that we are in need of radical improvement – assumed that we were insufficient for this world; that without a God that could keep us in mind – a God who, in however inscrutable a sense, knew what was going on – we were bereft and impoverished (and compared with an omniscient deity, or magically potent deities, we were indeed lacking). If mortality was a flaw, or a punishment, we were always verging on humiliation. Tyrannical fantasies of our own perfectibility still lurk in even our simplest ideals, Darwin and Freud intimate, so that any ideal can become another excuse for punishment. Lives dominated by impossible ideals – complete honesty, absolute knowledge, perfect happiness, eternal love – are lives experienced as continuous failure.

And yet people's capacity to survive, one way or

another, loss and even devastation is at once a banal and remarkable fact. Whether we talk of their resilience, their faith in their ideals, their opportunism or even their masochism, we can't help but be amazed by what people can live through. Though this hardiness is always at a cost, the sheer stubbornness of the so-called will to live is often cause for celebration, though quite what is being celebrated isn't always quite so clear, especially in a secular culture. Without a divine sanction to their lives – without a deity or deities to placate or impress – what self-justifying stories can people tell themselves, in order to keep going? This was the crisis of faith, in both their religions, that Darwin and Freud were born into as men of the nineteenth century; all the questions around what Ford Madox Ford referred to in 1924 as 'that mystic word "justification"'. In their writings we see religious traditions and sensibilities struggling to transform themselves into secular, scientifically informed ways of life. The new world of late-nineteenth-century Europe was a world possibly without God, not one that was closer to his divine purposes.

Both Darwin and Freud were fascinated by losses that could be survived – or even seen to be sources of inspiration – and by what survived, as evidence, of lives that had been lived. It was to these formative scenes of loss that they returned again and again in their writings. What could be made of what hadn't yet disappeared – the fossil record, or the half-remembered dream, species of birds or childhood memories – was their inspiration. It was the transience of things, the impermanence of natural phenomena, that fed them their best lines. Life was about what could be done with what was left, with what still happened to be there.

And this sophisticated scavenging that their theories were – and that their theories were about – foisted certain irrepressible questions upon them. Since a natural world is a world of continuous change and therefore continuous loss, how and why does loss matter? What kind of morality is apt in a world without divine sanction, and in which change is rife? What kind of loss or change is death itself, and what can it possibly mean to us in a secular world (our sadness may be just a bad old habit)? What can we say about death if we don't imagine what a god might be saying about it? If our new natural lives, our newly naturalized lives, were not to be a protracted mourning – an increasingly realistic and accurate acknowledgement of loss in its various guises – new pleasures had to be shored against our ruins. The risk was that life could be seen as an enormous waste; the pain of existence would not only be without justification, it could be without compensation.

And yet what is striking about Darwin's and Freud's work is that these different scenes of loss that they keep returning to are, more often than not, an occasion, an opportunity, for invention. Indeed these particular scenes make invention imperative. They are places to go on from, situations in which a good story must be told (though these stories can be an uneasy mixture of whistling in the dark and science). In other words, neither man is silenced by what he discovers, or finds himself making up. 'One *is* mortal,' Leslie Farber wrote, 'and since, by definition, mortality is crumbling, its claims are imperious.' And one of its claims now, in the work of Darwin and Freud, was to make unredeemed mortality itself more than merely bearable; to render ageing, accident, illness and death not alien but integral to our sense of ourselves; to find out whether loss is still the right word. That we might consider ourselves diminished by acknowledging, or even enjoying, such things – such things as time and bodily life – is a mark of just how distracted we have been. Believing there is a better world elsewhere now looks like a way of not seeing the sufficiencies of this one.

If there are no 'higher things', then there are no lower ones either. If anything unites Darwin and Freud it is a shrewd scepticism about what have traditionally been considered higher things. So they both recycle what their cultures try to disown and devalue and trivialize. And they do this, above all, by redescribing scenes of loss from a secular point of view. They want to show – both through their own performances in their writing, and through what they are actually describing – how and why people and other animals don't give up. Not merely how they avoid despair, though this is often lurking, but rather how they turn things to account; not so much the profit of loss, but its boon.

Darwin was always struck by the ingenious opportunism – always in the service of survival and reproduction – of the creatures he studied. They often seemed to have, by nature as it were, a genius for adaptation; until, that is, the environment finally became too much for them. There was always the possibility of being at a loss. 'I have as much difficulty as ever in expressing myself clearly and concisely,' Darwin wrote in his autobiography:

and this difficulty has caused me a very great loss of time: but it has had the compensating advantage of forcing me to think long and intently about every sentence, and thus I have been often led to see errors in reasoning and in my own observations or those of others. There seems to be a sort of fatality in my mind leading me to put at first my statement and proposition in a wrong or awkward form.

By losing time Darwin gained something else; it is because his efficient wished-for competence breaks down – he cannot immediately write as he would want to, clearly and concisely – that something else comes through, a different kind of attentiveness. His error – the wrong and awkward forms his writing takes at first – becomes his gift. It was the losses of time that he would write about, and that would enable him to write. In his writing habits Darwin finds himself doing something that creates a sense of loss; as though that experience of loss, of the waste of time, were itself a kind of source, ironically, of more life, of better sentences. The obstacle proves to be the instrument, the loss is a calling. He is writing about how he has gone on writing. It is indeed a 'very great loss of time', because it has provided him, and us, with so many good sentences. He had to lose time in order to find something else. This losing is an art; it inspires a new quality of attention.

When Freud observed how his one-and-a-half-year-old grandson dealt with the loss of his mother, he was impressed by the child's inventiveness; the way the child transformed the mother's absence into a pleasurable game. 'The child had a wooden reel with a piece of string tied round it,' Freud wrote in *Beyond the Pleasure Principle*:

> What he did was to hold the reel by the string and very skilfully throw it over the edge of his curtained cot, so that it disappeared into it, at the same time uttering his expressive 'o-o-o-o'. He then pulled the reel out of the cot again by the string and hailed its reappearance with a joyful 'da' (there). This, then, was the complete game – disappearance and return. As a rule one only witnessed its first act, which was repeated untiringly as a game in itself, though there is no doubt that the greater pleasure was attached to the second act. The interpretation of the game then became obvious. It was related to the child's great cultural achievement – the instinctual renunciation ... which he had made in allowing his mother to go away without protesting. He compensated himself for this, as it were, by himself staging the disappearance and return of the objects within his reach.

Without the invention of this game, one might think, the child would feel the unbearable pain of his mother's absence. And yet as Freud describes this scene – in which for him too the woman, his daughter, is absent; and in which he too makes up a story – it is not as though the child is merely making a choice to manage his suffering, but rather that the mother's absence is an opportunity for the child to find another pleasure. And not only the ascetic pleasure of instinctual renunciation, but the pleasure of symbolization itself; the delight of making up the game. Whether or not loss is being mastered by the child – whatever that might mean – a new talent is being found; and being found to be so pleasurable that it is repeated, 'untiringly, as a game in itself'. The situation calls up something new in the child. Without the mother's absence there would have been no game, no new pleasure nor Freud's new theory (just as, without Darwin's very great loss of time, there would not have been his best sentences). And what the child discovers is that he can now have two pleasures for the price of one: this child still has a mother, and he has acquired a new game for himself; and he can have both (if not always at the same time). All Freud's language – the child 'very skilfully' throwing the reel, his 'expressive', 'joyful' sounds, the child's 'great cultural achievement' – celebrates the child as artist, discovering his artistry; and not merely (or bitterly) actively re-enacting with his toys what he has had unavoidably inflicted on him.

'When it plays at "throwing things far away",' Moustafa Safouan writes, 'the child is trying out this new freedom.' This particular new freedom – to live well in the absence of the mother, to make and take things up – is only available to the child when the mother goes away. Compensation may be the wrong word here (as for Darwin); what Freud and Darwin actually describe – and Freud is also, by implication, writing about writing here – is more akin to the artful elaboration of an experience. The child, after all, is not finding a substitute for the mother, because there isn't one, but an extension of her (something comforting and pleasurable) that is also an alternative to her. More of the same – mother all the time – would spell the death of innovation. What is it inside us, Freud seems to be wondering, that can turn an absence into a pleasurably open space, that makes an improvisation out of a deprivation?

Of course the child must know somewhere, by now, that the game too could disappear (the reel could be taken away from him, just like the mother is). But the new 'skill' the child might acquire in the mother's absence is this very talent for dealing with albeit temporary disappearances. The child, that is to say, is learning the arts of transience. And he must learn that loss – hopefully not more than he can actually bear – is a permanent presence in life. Indeed, in Freud's view, this will be the child's most absorbing task; and especially when it comes to the real death of loved ones.

In what he calls, in *Mourning and Melancholia*, 'normal mourning' a person

> overcomes the loss of the object, and it, too, while it lasts, absorbs all the energies of the ego ... Each single one of the memories and situations of expectancy which demonstrate the libido's attachment

to the lost object is met by the verdict of reality that the object no longer exists; and the ego, confronted, as it were with the question whether it shall share this fate, is persuaded by the sum of the narcissistic satisfactions it derives from being alive to sever its attachment to the object that has been abolished.

So-called normal mourning is possible, Freud says, because eventually the mourner prefers more life to more death. But it is, as he puts it, a question; the fate of being alive has to be deemed more satisfying than the fate of being dead. The mourner, like the child in the game, Freud hopes, will choose life. 'The fact is,' he writes with unprecedented (and improbable) optimism, 'that when the work of mourning is completed the ego becomes free and uninhibited again.' Since, in Freud's view, the ego is and was never free and uninhibited, this is clearly Freud's wish: that normal mourning – what I am calling acknowledgement of transience – should be a release and a benefit. It should, like the child's game, free us for something, which is, among other things, the ongoing experience of transience. Freud, of course, never takes suffering out of the picture – 'It is remarkable,' Freud remarks, 'that this painful unpleasure (of mourning) is taken as a matter of course by us' – but he too, like the successful mourner in whom he invests his belief, takes it as a matter of course.

In both these examples there is what John Cage referred to as 'just the right amount of suffering';

neither Darwin nor Freud's grandson was paralysed or embittered by what he had to endure. They were ultimately inspired, and therefore reassured. Indeed the implied paradox, if we were to generalize from these two reports, would be: sometimes we suffer most from being unwilling to suffer enough. Darwin could have given up on expressing himself, just as the child can only find his game (and the new self that plays it) by first acknowledging the mother's absence. But something beyond what is traditionally called will-power is required of them; these are situations in which will-power won't work. So one of the defining scenarios for Darwin and Freud – the drama that organized their sentences – was of the person at a loss. What had previously been described in theological terms – as the presence or absence of God – was seeking its secular counterpart. And it is the simplest, most mundane of experiences: something that is wanted not being there (Darwin's best, most accurate sentences; the child's mother; Freud wanting a good story to explain the child's behaviour). And then the impossibility of it being willed into existence.

If the death of loved or needed people was always too stark an example of this fundamental experience, one's own death was the most imaginatively confounding one. It is as though, whatever else they are, all the quotidian experiences of loss, all the disappearances of everyday life, are like rehearsals, or conjectures, or foreshadowings: ironic speculations about the hidden drama of one's own death; getting in practice for one's own absence. Memory, and the reconstruction of histories, are so important to Darwin and Freud because they are our ordinary way of talking about our primal, initiating relationship to loss. People may die and be remembered; but they only disappear when they are completely forgotten, when no one ever uses their name. It is obvious why a child, or indeed an adult, would fear being forgotten; it is less clear why we fear forgetting the dead. Not forgetting, in other words, is, in Glenda Fredman's phrase, death-talk.

Writing about the fact that (in a very similar way to the forgetting of names) 'distressing memories succumb especially easily to motivated forgetting' Freud, in *The Psychopathology of Everyday Life*, invokes Darwin. 'The great Darwin,' Freud writes, 'laid down a "golden rule" for the scientific worker based on his insight into the part played by unpleasure as a motive for forgetting'; and Freud then quotes in a footnote something from Darwin's *Autobiography* which, in his view, 'convincingly reflects his scientific honesty and his psychological acumen', two things that for Freud tended to go together:

> I had, during many years, followed a golden rule, namely, that whenever a published fact, a new observation or thought came across me, which was opposed to my general results, to make a memorandum of it without fail and at once; for I had found by experience that such facts and thoughts were far more apt to escape from the memory than favourable ones.

An autobiography, of course, like a biography, is the remembering that is intended to remind other people (Darwin wrote his *Autobiography*, he said, for his family). One is, Darwin suggests here, more likely to forget what is disagreeable to oneself, but what is most disagreeable may be of most value. Once again, and like Freud, Darwin is awake to and alerted by what is likely to disappear (and the notion of a thought coming across him is itself suggestive). We are not only the victims of transience – the temporariness of our lives and the lives of others foisted upon us – we are also its agents. As part of nature, we inflict it on things. Organisms are creatures who rid themselves of things, of whatever is sufficiently painful, and therefore dangerous. And the art of life, or perhaps the art of science, is in being able to tell good riddance from bad. Because loss is endemic, retrieval is essential, 'without fail and at once'. The scientific method, as described by Darwin and endorsed here by Freud, staves off entropy. But this retrieval that is a form of memory is good, not because it wishfully stops time – monumentalizes the past – but because, in their view, it sponsors change. And being able or willing to change is, in the strongest sense, adaptive. As though what was unbearable for people was the sheer voraciousness of change. The new Darwinian or Freudian person – born and growing up in the newfound flourish and terror of a mercilessly expansive capitalism – had to be committed to instability. It was, unsurprisingly, economies of loss, in their secular versions, that preoccupied Darwin and Freud.

At a time when profit, in its increasingly less various guises, was becoming the cultural idol, the capital they wanted to accumulate was scientific knowledge of the past. There were profits to be made – and Darwin, like his family before him, was an investor – but losses were always incurred. There was always, that is to say, the paltry fact: that money doesn't make death or the vulnerability of the body disappear from the horizon. It was to write about loss without writing about despair – without the refuge of optimism, the confidence of nihilism, or the omniscience of the tragic view – that had become the challenge.

Darwin will record his falsifying evidence, like the patient in analysis recuperating (and recuperating from) their distressing memories, so that it can eventually and finally disappear into his own more convincing formulations. Darwin and Freud, that is to say, in their quite different ways are persuading us to become good losers; to be able, if need be, to dispel our attachment to people and ideas, and ultimately to ourselves. It is as though, they suggest, we have added to the ordinary suffering of biological life the extraordinary suffering of our immortal longings, of our will to permanence. As though our equating of value with duration over time – good relationships, like great art are the ones that last: truths are eternal essences amid the ruinous wastes of time, and so on – straightforwardly turns a blind eye to all the evidence. As though there has always been the unbearable fact of impermanence, and all our solutions to this abiding fact can seem like evasions; there is the Scylla of nostalgia and the Charybdis of dread. The writings of Darwin and Freud, above all perhaps, make us wonder quite why this is such intolerable knowledge, so that it can often be glibly referred to, without our ever being able to live as though it were really true. If it has been the tendency of at least Western belief systems to value what is immortal – God, Truth, the Soul – Darwin and Freud encourage us to describe what this craving for continuities might be a solution to. And they press us to think of our lives as more miraculous than our deaths; our death is inevitable, but our conception is not.

Belief in what was once called the perfectibility of man – and might now be called cure or normality or success – their writing suggests, destroys our hopes for (and in) this world. Our ideals baffle and conceal our possibilities; the very falsity of our hopes inevitably defeats us. For Freud biography – with its aspiration, or even its claim, to provide an authoritative or in any way truthful account *from outside* of a person's life – was a spurious and misleading idea (there can be no substitute, as psychoanalysis showed, for a person's own account of her life). The mystery of a life, its stubborn secretive intents, was best captured by the fiction of a death instinct, and the supreme fiction of an unconscious ('The unconscious is the true psychical reality,' Freud wrote in *The Interpretation of Dreams*, 'in its innermost nature it is as much unknown to us as the reality of the external world.'). Our knowledge claims, in other words, are always in question, if not intrinsically self-deceiving. For Darwin the whole notion of co-operation or collaboration – of anything akin to altruism – *beyond a certain point* was a version of that disabling perfectionism called Christianity that flew in the face of the evidence. Darwin's facts may have been subject to revision, but there was no getting away from them. Like his favoured worms, organisms might happen to collaborate with each other and even with other species (even if this could not be described as their intention); but their survival in order to reproduce would always set ineluctable limits to the very real communality that could be observed to exist in nature.

In Darwin's and Freud's view it was our relentless, unforgiving attachment to the available varieties of perfectionism – to idealizing our ideals – that consistently humiliated us. There was a will to pessimism in our choosing spurious, impossible ideals for ourselves; as though we had somehow become addicted to looking disappointing in our own eyes. We had diminished ourselves from our own too closely guarded point of view. We could only idealize our ideals because we were caught up in two false beliefs, the belief in redemption (and its secular equivalents perfect happiness, total knowledge, cure), and the belief that we could stop time (find some way of exempting ourselves, of excusing ourselves from change). It was the art of being realistic optimists – but neither depressed, nor cynical, nor unduly narcissistic – that Darwin and Freud wanted to interest us in: the worm and not the biographer. The only world that is possible must be the best of all possible worlds.

'Men are called "creatures of reason",' Darwin wrote in his Notebook in 1839; 'more appropriately they would be "creatures of habit".' Habit is evidence of adaptation, but habits are disabling when they tacitly assume that the future will be like the past. Our survival in what is always a changing environment depends upon our capacity to change our habits if need be. Habit, like bad science (or prejudice), creates an illusion of predictability; it keeps things the same by turning a blind eye to difference. We don't reason, Darwin suggests, we familiarize; we don't look for (or easily bear) the unknown, we assume a knowingness. Science, for Darwin like survival itself, involves us acquiring a paradoxical, a painful pleasure: the pleasure of having our previously held habitual beliefs disconfirmed, an eagerness to recognize our most deeply cherished untruths. And all this, becoming the creatures of real reason, means simply: being alert to what is actually going on around us. Every time we are able to relinquish a false conviction – a habit rather than a reasonable belief, in Darwin's language – we connect ourselves to the world. Untruths begin to look like refuges, spurious forms of self-isolation. Change – 'dear to all things not to themselves endeared', in Randall Jarrell's words – is always there waiting to be moralized (as loss, progress, purpose, waste); it is the fact about which, out of which, we weave our fictions. Habit is the opposite of reason for

Darwin because it can keep us out of time with ourselves.

Freud's word for habits was symptoms. If mourning was the most emotionally vivid example of what it was to change one's habits, symptoms were by definition – by the fact of their repetition – holding operations; ways of living in the present by holding on to the past. What Freud added to Darwin's belief in adaptation – the ongoing process of conformity and innovation – was the idea of our having to adapt to what he called the internal world (of desires, and prohibitions, and memory). Externally *and* internally, the struggle goes on to turn unruliness into habit, waywardness into familiarity. Freud's therapeutic 'method' of free association was invented, if not merely to cure people of their (unwanted) habits, at least to reveal what they might be, and what they are used to do. 'Instead of urging the patient', Freud writes in his *An Autobiographical Study*,

> to say something on some particular subject, I now asked him to abandon himself to the process of *free association* – that is, to say whatever came into his head, while ceasing to give any conscious direction to his thoughts. It was essential, however, that he should bind himself to report literally everything that occurred to his self-perception and not to give way to critical objections which sought to put certain associations on one side on the ground that they were not sufficiently important or that they were irrelevant or that they were altogether meaningless.

There are, in other words, things that come into our heads that it is our habit to dismiss; through which, in all this abandoning and binding of himself – this newish discipline that sounds strangely like a sexual practice in Freud's description – the 'patient' can gain access to something vital. And by being better adapted – in the sense of responsive to and accommodating of – to the vagaries of his internal world the patient will be better adapted to his external world. Purposive thinking, a too lucid sense of the task, what Freud calls 'urging the patient to say something upon some particular subject', paradoxically limits the available information; just as the foreground of a picture can render the background that has made it possible invisible. To free-associate the patient has to give up many of his previous attachments: his attachment to his more familiar thoughts and habitual associations, his attachment to being acceptable (or loveable) to the person in whose presence he speaks, his attachment to recognizing the self he knows in the words he speaks; his attachment, above all, perhaps, to the idea that there is some particular subject about which he can speak. Free-associating, that is to say, is akin to mourning; it is a process of detachment that releases hidden energies.

The new world of continuous change – the daunting new world that Darwin and Freud both report back from and inaugurate with their distinctive descriptions – is a world of continuous loss. And yet neither Darwin nor Freud in his writings is grief-stricken (despite the fact, for example, that both men lost, among other people in their lives, their favourite daughters). They perform in their writings an intrigued resilience, neither bumptiously optimistic nor complacently gloomy. While they aspire to the dispassionate plausibility of their scientific genres, they can avoid turning their various knowledges of the past into forms of unremitting elegy. Their catalogues of loss are records also of survival; indeed, this is what makes evidence of the past so inspiring for them. And they can relish the new – whatever is still here and changing – because it represents the ingenuities of its own endurance. And it is part of their being impressed by the advantages of life that they cannot help occasionally giving us tips along the way about what seems to work.

Darwin, who had even less therapeutic (that is, prophetic) intent than Freud, wanted to share, in his calmly understated way, his own observations about the 'lower' forms of life. 'When there exists an inherited or instinctive tendency to the performance of an action, or an inherited taste for certain kinds of food,' he wrote in *The Expression of the Emotions in Man and Animals*,

> some degree of habit in the individual is often or generally requisite ... Caterpillars which have been fed on the leaves of one kind of tree, have been known to perish from hunger rather than to eat the leaves of another tree, although this afforded them their proper food, under a state of nature; and so it is in many other cases. The power of association is admitted by everyone.

The habits that sustain us can be deadly; it is we, in Darwin's characteristically quiet irony, that are among the many other cases. If we, like other creatures can prefer our habits to our lives – if we love our routines more than our futures – then we are fatally addicted to the past. Sometimes our old, habitual associations need to be turned into looser ends. In showing us the paradoxical subtleties of adaptation even in the most apparently rudimentary organisms, or the point of free association and 'ordinary mourning', Darwin and Freud are promoting, above all, the (survival-) value of mobility (the unconscious, like the ecosystem, is full of fast moves and old habits). There is something bright about the opportunism, or lack of it, that both of them keep noticing in the creatures that interest them (the diligent caterpillar, like the obsessional person, is undernourished, at the deadest of ends). They describe, or implicitly prescribe, the intelligence (the reason) of certain kinds of promiscuity – in the individual constructing his dream, or the successful species exploiting its niche – but without asking us to give up on history, and therefore on loyalties and allegiances from the past. The past is not the kind of thing that for them could ever be abandoned; it can only be variously reconstructed and experienced. And though they both temper their stories and histories and hypotheses with evidence, as they must – the burden of proof, as traditionally conceived, being rather more of a problem for Freud than for Darwin – exhilaration keeps bursting through in their writing. And it is the exhilaration, however banal it might sound, of loving nature. But they have to re-invent love because nature for them is not an idol (neither a mother nor a father nor a god). Whether it is the heroic romance of worms or the ironic questings of a putative death instinct, their writing has all the inspiring persistence, the uncanny ingeniousness, of their nominal subjects (they are also, in other words, all the time finding analogies for their own imaginative activities). Darwin is as patiently thorough, as profoundly industrious as his worms: Freud is as intent and sly as his death instinct.

And yet what they both counsel is often at once beguilingly simple – even if its consequences are not – and peculiarly puzzling. They ask us to believe in the permanence only of change and uncertainty: that the only life is the life of the body, so that death, in whatever form it takes, is of a piece with life. When Darwin writes about his talented worms, or Freud writes about his shrewd, wayward death instinct, they are presenting us with new kinds of heroic nature. And by doing so they ask us, ultimately, to imagine ourselves, to describe ourselves from nature's point of view; but in the full knowledge that nature, by (their) definition, doesn't have one. They want us, in short, not to be unduly dismayed by our mortality – to live with our own deaths.

Acknowledgements

A version of 'Darwin Turns The Worm' was published in *Raritan*. I am grateful as ever for the enthusiastic interest of the editors of that journal, Richard Poirier and Suzanne Hyman. Hugh Haughton, Cora Kaplan, Hermione Lee and John Forrester invited me to present parts of this book at (respectively) the universities of York, Southampton, Oxford and Cambridge. Their comments, and the audience discussions, significantly changed my sense of what I was doing. Jacqueline Rose, Kate Weaver, Geoffrey Weaver, and Felicity Rubenstein were essential first readers. Jacqueline Rose also did some crucial translating.

Bibliography

Janet Browne, *Charles Darwin, Voyaging* (London, Pimlico, 1995)

Charles Darwin, *Formation of Vegetable Mould Through the Action of Worms, with Observations on their Habits (1881)* (Chicago, Chicago University Press, 1985)

The Origin of Species (Oxford, Oxford University Press, 1986)

The Collected Papers of Charles Darwin, edited by Paul H. Barrett (Chicago, Chicago University Press, 1977)

The Expression of the Emotions in Man and Animals (London, Harper Collins, 1998)

Metaphysics, Materialism and the Evolution of Mind, Early writings of Charles Darwin (Chicago, Chicago University Press, 1974)

The Correspondence of Charles Darwin, Vol. 2, edited by Frederick Burckhardt and Sidney Smith (Cambridge, Cambridge University Press, 1986)

Charles Darwin's Letters, A Selection, edited by Frederick Burckhardt (Cambridge, Cambridge University Press, 1996)

Autobiography (Oxford, Oxford University Press, 1974)

Adrian Desmond and James Moore, *Darwin* (London, Michael Joseph, 1991)

Richard Dawkins, *The Selfish Gene* (Oxford, Oxford University Press, 1989)

Deleuze and Guattari, *Anti-Oedipus*, translated by Robert Hurley (London, The Athlone Press, 1983)

Leslie Farber, *Lying, Despair, Jealousy, Envy, Sex, Suicide, Drugs and the Good Life* (New York, Basic Books, 1976)

Ford Madox Ford, *Josesph Conrad: A Personal Remembrance* (New York, Ecco Press, 1989)

Glenda Fredman, *Death Talk* (London, Karnak Books, 1997)

Anna Freud, *Selected Writings*, edited by Richard Ekins and Ruth Freeman (London, Penguin Books, 1998)

Sigmund Freud, *The Standard Edition of the Complete Psychological Works of Sigmund Freud*, ed. and trans. James Strachey (London, Hogarth Press, 1953–74)

The Letters of Sigmund Freud and Arnold Zweig, edited by Ernst L. Freud (London, Hogarth Press, 1970)

Letters of Sigmund Freud, 1873–1939, edited by Ernst L. Freud (London, Hogarth Press, 1960)

Peter Gay, *Freud* (London, Macmillan, 1988)

Stephen Jay Gould, *Life's Grandeur* (London, Jonathan Cape, 1996)

Randall Jarrell, 'Children Selecting Books in the Library', in *The Complete Poems* (London, Faber and Faber, 1971)

Ernest Jones, *Sigmund Freud, Life and Work*, Vol. III (London, Hogarth Press, 1957)

Frank Kermode, *The Sense of an Ending* (Oxford, Oxford University Press, 1967)

Jacques Lacan *The Statutes proposed by Jacques Lacan for the Institute of Psychoanalysis 1953: La Scission de 1953* (trans. J. Rose)

Jean Laplanche, *Essays on Otherness*, edited by John Fletcher (London, Routledge, 1999)

Philip Larkin, *Collected Poems* (London, Faber, 1988)

J.-B. Pontalis, *Frontiers in Psychoanalysis* (London, Hogarth Press, 1981)

Ruth Anna Putnam, 'The Moral Impulse' in *The Revival of Pragmatism*, edited by Morris Dickstein (Durham, Duke University Press, 1998)

Moustapha Safouan, *Pleasure and Being*, trans. by Martin Thom (London, Macmillan, 1983)

William Shakespeare, *Hamlet*, edited by Harold Jenkins (London, Methuen, 1982)

Wallace Stevens, *Collected Poetry & Prose*, edited by Frank Kermode and Joan Richardson (New York, The Library of America, 1997)

Lionel Trilling, *Freud and the Crisis of our Culture* (Boston, Beacon Press, 1955)

BIBLIOGRAPHY

Tennyson, *A Selected Edition*, ed. Christopher Ricks (London, Longman, 1989)

Thomas Weiskel, *The Romantic Sublime* (Baltimore, Johns Hopkins University Press, 1976)

Raymond Williams, *Keywords*, (London, Fontana, 1976)

Index

145